ISO-BOW
POWER PUMP
WORKOUTS II

ISO-BOW POWER PUMP

WORKOUTS II

The Best Isotonic method that build muscle mass, increase power, and sculpt your best body Today!

The Iso-Bow Power Pump Workouts II was written to help you get closer to your physical potential when it comes to real muscle sculpting strengthening exercises. The exercises and routines in this book are quite demanding, so consult your physician and have a physical exam taken prior to the start of this exercise program. Proceed with the suggested exercises and information at your own risk. The Publishers and author shall not be liable or responsible for any loss, injury, or damage allegedly arising from the information or suggestions in this book.

Iso-Bow Power Pump Workouts II
muscle-building Course

By

Birch Tree Publishing
Published by Birch Tree Publishing

Iso-Bow Power Pump Workouts II
Published in 2020, All rights reserved,
No part of this book may be reproduced, scanned,
or distributed in any printed or electronic form without permission.

Birch Tree Publishing

Dedication

Bullworker fans, here's book four to the ISO-BOW **POWER PUMP SERIES**

Contents

BUILD MUSCLES FAST!

With the worlds fastest physique enhancing series

Introduction by John Hughes

I have been involved with athletics all of my life, from college wrestling to World Championship Master's Wrestling in my 60s. Coupled with over 15 years of high school coaching, I have always strived for top physical performance in strength and flexibility for myself and the athletes I coached. I purchased my first Bullworker in the 1960s and was impressed with how quickly my body responded to Bullworker strength training. The portability of the product meant I never had to get rid of it due to space restraints and over the next 30 years, the ability to supplement any exercise routine with a quick Bullworker workout, always complimented my desired fitness goal.

In 1999, I became the North American distributor for Bullworker and began to work on design changes to make the product much more challenging, yet always maintaining the portability aspect of this time tested and proven fitness product. In recognizing the importance of cross-training principles for maximum fitness results, I designed additional products that kept with the Bullworker portability concept with each product able to be used either separately or combined for maximum fitness results in a complete cross-training program.

In 2010, I purchased most of the Global rights to Bullworker and have reintroduced Bullworker training principles that have been effective since 1962 and resulted in over 10 million units sold. Proven as the ultimate portable fitness products, Bullworker continues to deliver results to everyone, any age, wherever they exercise.

Now, I present the Iso-Bow Power Series. This book is about transforming your body, mind and spirit, which is what health, strength and physique enhancement is all about. I am really excited and positive to say that once you try the programs in this book, you will make some of the best gains you've ever made.

Join the men and women that are already using The Bullworker Power Series and programs with great success. **GET TRANSFORMED** today.

Keep pulling and pushing

Yours in Strength and Power
John Hughes

ISO-BOW STRONG!

LET'S GO

If you are reading this book, you already appreciate the importance of exercising for health, strength and wellbeing. The Power Iso-Bow Transformation Method will turn you into a powerful well built man. Being a great success at exercising means constant practice to transform yourself to become the best you can be.

When it comes to training-like most everything else in life-sometimes circumstances seem to get in the way from allowing you to exercise. Now, thanks to The Power Iso-Bow Method, you will always get a great workout-no matter where you are.

Resistance strength training with The Power Iso-Bow Method enhances:

1) Resistance strength training stimulates muscles to burn more calories than anything else. After your workout your metabolism is triggered for 40 hours after the session.
2) Your body will take on a different shape, and your clothes will fit far better.
3) Your flexibility will increase and resistance training will keep you young.
4) Your bones will become stronger. We lose bone mass as we get older, but resistance strength training increases bone density and add greater strength.
5) A stronger and healthy heart with enhanced blood flow.
6) Stress levels will be reduced due to exercise.
7) Resistance strength training also creates better sleeping patterns.
8) "No need to get depressed". Regular resistance training will ward off symptoms of depression.
9) Mental sharpness will be developed. This takes place due resistance training decreasing blood levels of homocysteine, the protein that's linked to developing Alzheimer's and dementia. Plus, resistance training enhances cognitive function. Workouts will improve memory and you will have longer attention spans.
10) Develop lazar-like focus.

The Training Series that will create a Powerful Iso-Bow Body

Chapter 1:
CHEST

Build a Powerful Chest

Create the body of your dreams with the Iso-Bow

Chapter 1:

CHEST

BUILD A POWERFUL CHEST

BUILD A POWERFUL CHEST

01 BUILD A POWERFUL CHEST

The chest muscles allow you to push or move the arm forward or across the body. These muscles are activated in any throwing or pushing motion. Aesthetically, building a powerful chest is a sign of power in men.

However, the chest muscles are not used daily, so most times they are under developed. So despite, the simplicity of how these muscles contract, they can be trained in a number of various angles of push and pull, each offer its own special muscle enhancing properties.

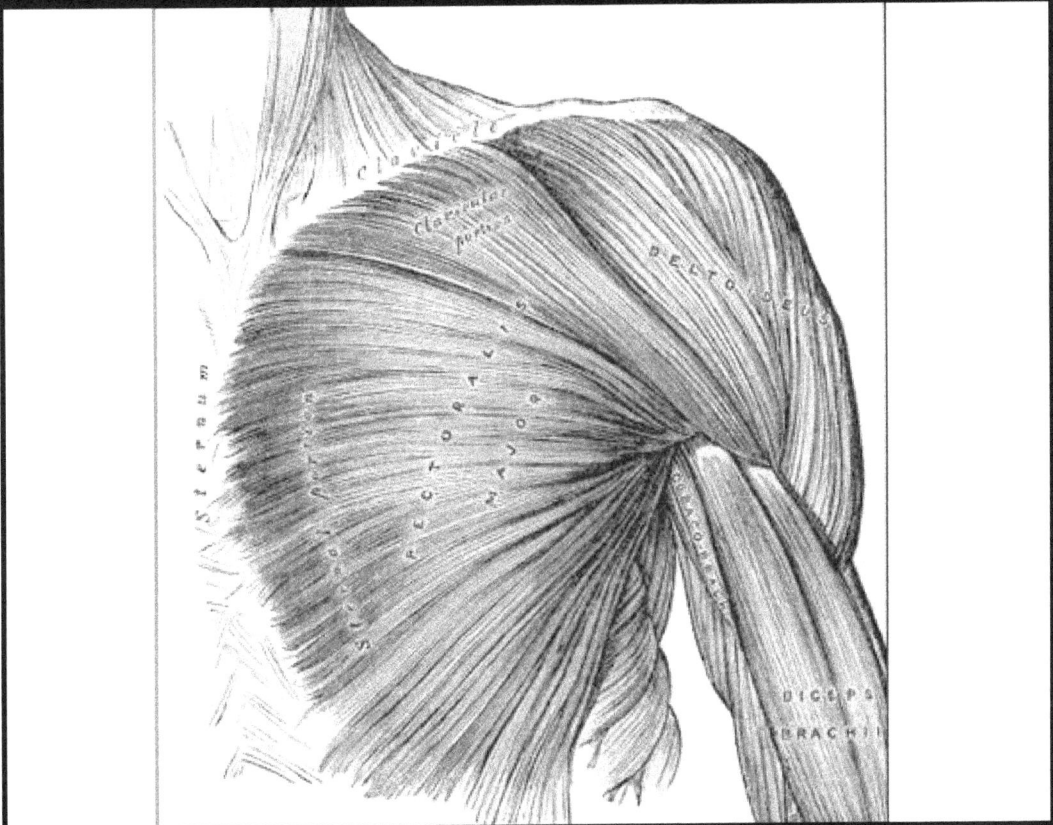

CHEST EXERCISES

01 BUILD A POWERFUL CHEST

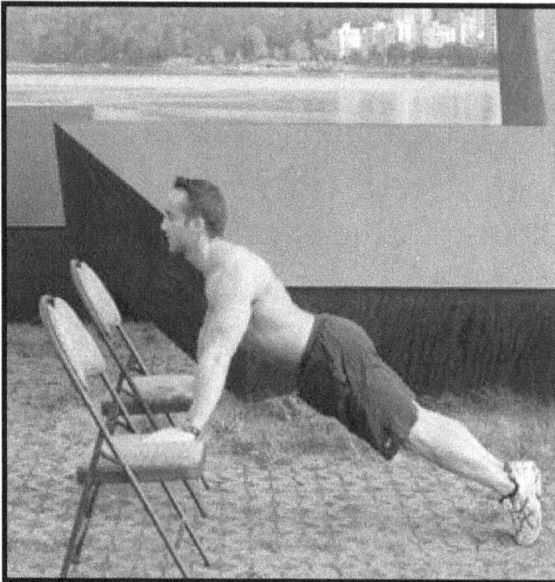

INCLINE PUSHUPS

Place your hands on two chairs that are 15 inches high, the higher you go the greater pre-stretch there is. At the bottom position to enhance muscle-building stimuli, pause for 2 seconds before reversing the movement. This is an excellent warm up before your chest contraction exercises.

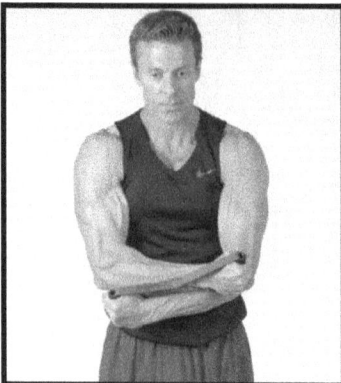

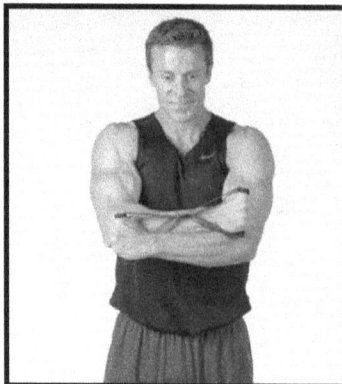

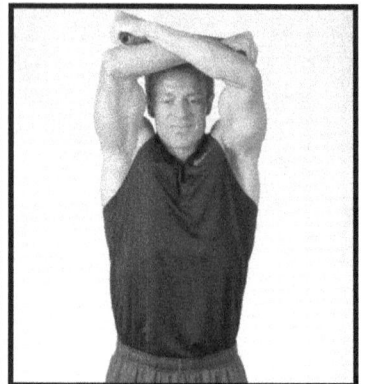

CHEST CONTRACTION

Cross arms as shown press the arms in opposite directions maintaining the tension. **(Isometric Contraction)** Now move your arm upwards and overhead, then reverse the motion maintaining strong tension. **DUAL ACTION**

Chapter 2:

SHOULDERS
DEVELOP POWERFUL SHOULDERS

DEVELOP POWERFUL SHOULDERS

02 DEVELOP POWERFUL SHOULDERS

The shoulder muscles are divided into three heads and are quite unique and move the arm in all directions. The front muscle raise the arm forward, the side muscles made up of a number of muscle bundles, and raises the arm out to the sides. The rear or posterior muscle, is designed to pull the arm backwards. Shoulder presses is a multi-muscle-use exercise, which is a compound exercise. This exercise recruits the front and side heads of the shoulders that tie in well with stimulating the upper and mid-back muscles as well giving the entire girdle complete development.

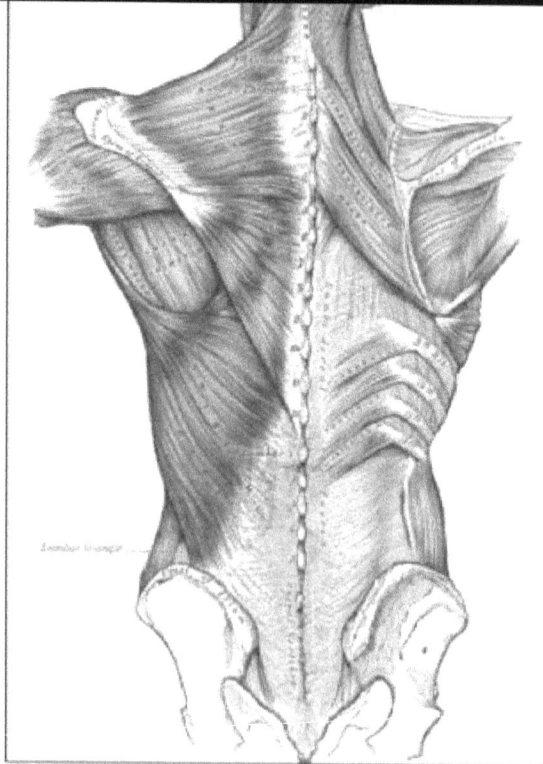

SHOULDER EXERCISES

02 DEVELOP POWERFUL SHOULDERS

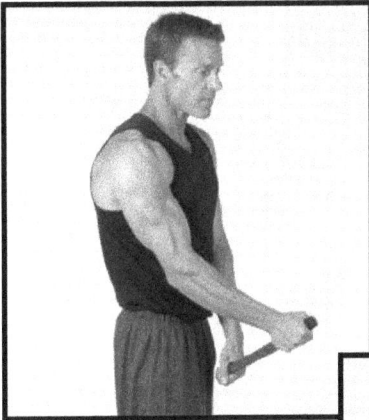

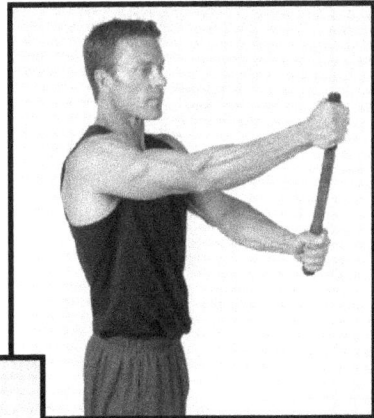

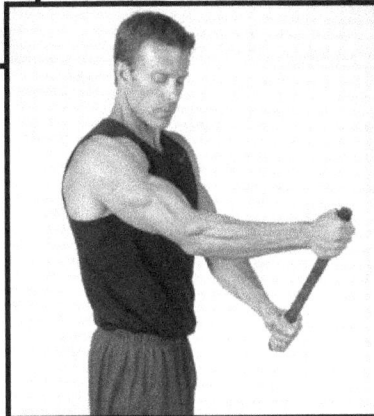

FORWARD RAISES

Grasp the Iso-Bow in front of the body, as shown. Gradually raise the arm forward against the resistance of the other hand. **RESIST IN THE UP MOTION ONLY** This works the front part of the shoulder muscles.

SHOULDER EXERCISES

02 DEVELOP BARN DOOR SHOULDERS

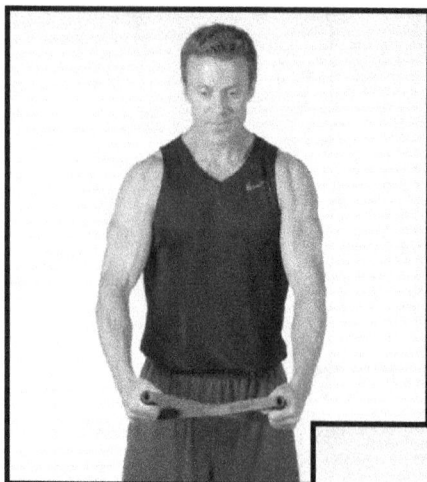

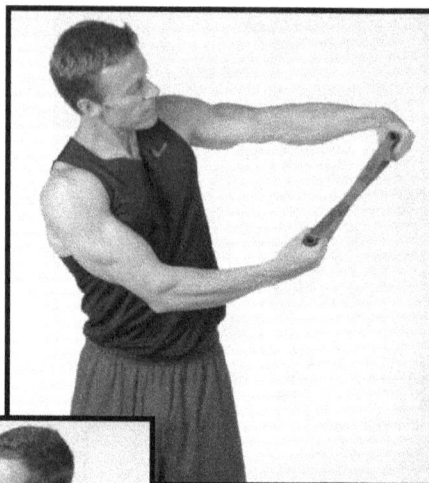

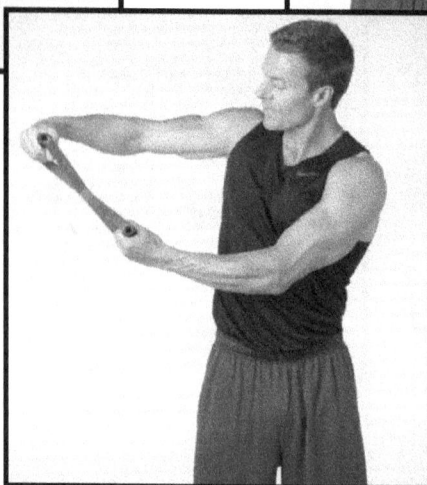

LATERAL RAISES

Hold the Iso-Bow at waist, keep your elbows slightly bent, raise your arm as shown while resisting with the other arm. Perform all reps on one side first before switching arms. **RESIST IN ONE DIRECTION ONLY**

SHOULDER EXERCISES

02 DEVELOP POWERFUL SHOULDERS

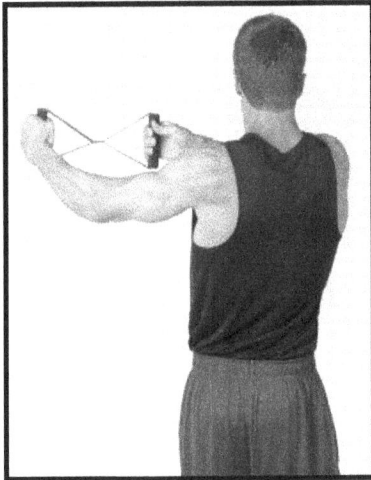

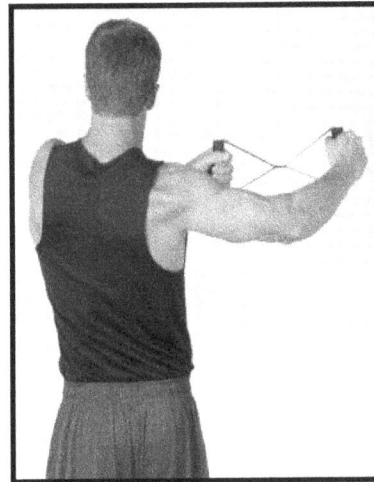

ACROSS THE BODY PULLS

Place the Iso-Bow at chest height, keep your elbows slightly bent, pull the arm toward the right while resisting with the other arm. Pause and reverse the motion alternating sides. **DUAL ACTION RESIST IN BOTH DIRECTIONS**

Chapter 3:

UPPER BACK
DEVELOP A POWERFUL V-TAPER

DEVELOP A POWERFUL V-TAPER

03 DEVELOP A POWERFUL V-TAPER

The entire back is made up of many muscles overlapping each other. However, most trainees find the back quite difficult to fully develop. The reason? As the saying goes out of sight, out of mind. We cannot directly see the back muscles, plus we cannot see it flex like we would see the biceps.

We make training the entire back musculature much easier making developing the back obviously simple once you know what you are doing, you can bring these muscles up to speed. We are looking at the large Latissimus that covers the majority of the back. The trapezius is broken up into two sections.

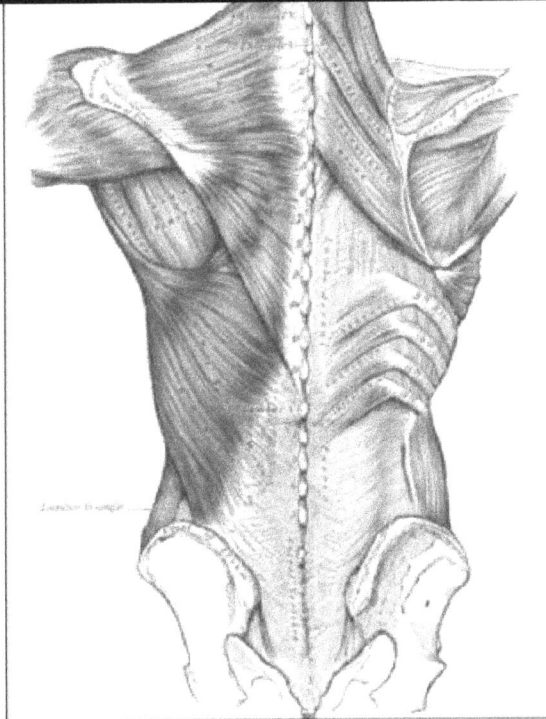

UPPER BACK EXERCISES

03 DEVELOP A POWERFUL V-TAPER

DO NOT NEGLECT THE MID AND LOWER TRAPS

The upper traps and mid-back muscles. Plus, we have the teres major, which is strongly stimulated with unilateral work, which makes self resistance the ideal movement. The infraspinatus muscle is like a half circle on each side of the upper back and is a very important rotator cuff muscle.

This muscle stabilizes the shoulder and prevents dislocations. Even though this muscle is at the back, most traditional exercises do not fully target these muscles. However, with self resistance there are exercises that target this area for full development.

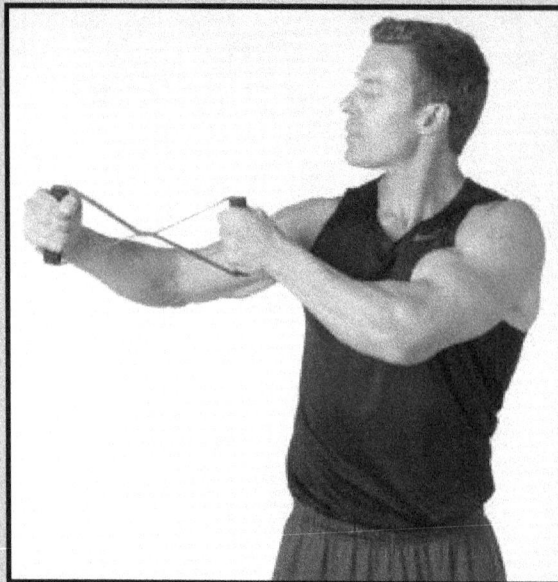

UPPER BACK EXERCISES

03 DEVELOP A POWERFUL V-TAPER

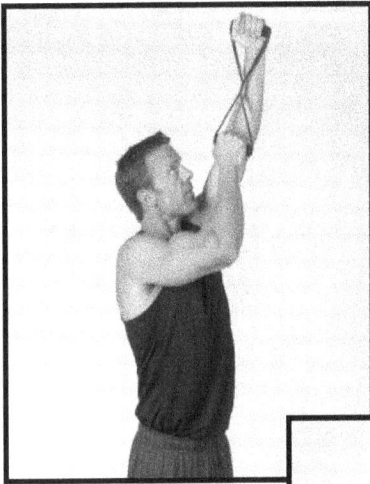

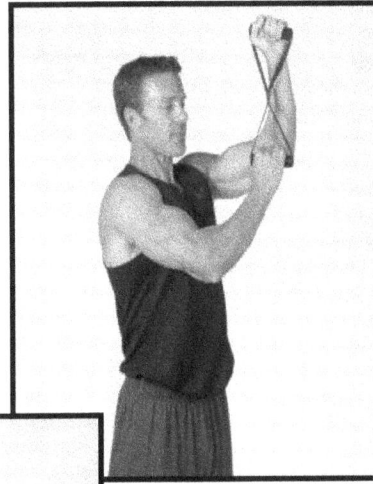

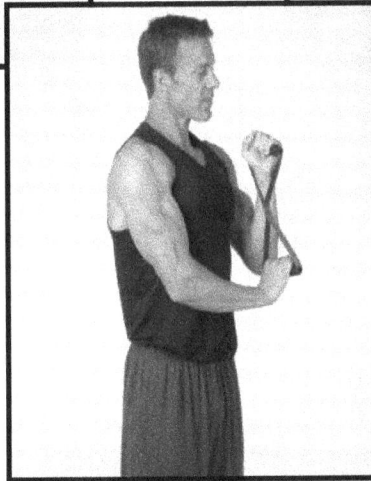

PULLDOWNS

Grasp the Iso-Bow as shown in the picture. Gradually pull the arm
downwards while resisting with the bottom arm. **RESIST IN ONE DIRECTION ONLY**

UPPER BACK EXERCISES

03 DEVELOP A POWERFUL V-TAPER

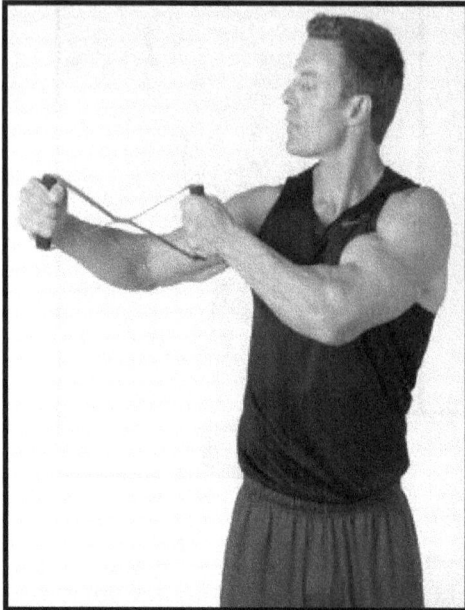

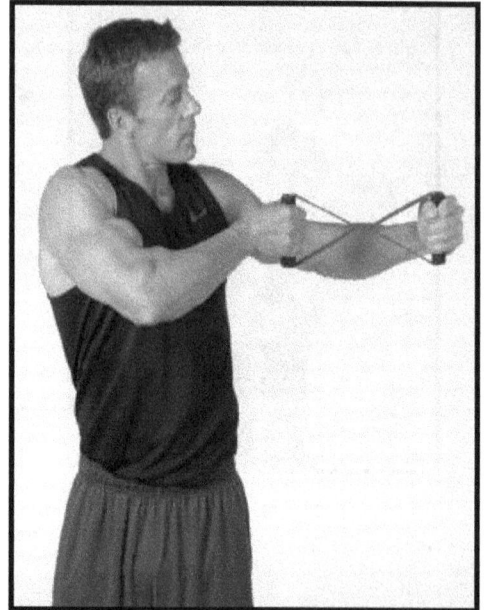

UPPER BACK ROWS

Bring your arm across the body pre-stretching the mid-back, grasp the Iso-Bow as shown. Slowly pull the arm across the body toward the armpit against the resistance supplied by the other arm. Extend the arm back to the starting position. Repeat the movement, then switch arms. This adds thickens to the mid-back, lats, and biceps along with the rear part of the shoulders.
RESIST IN A DUAL MANNER

UPPER BACK EXERCISES

03 DEVELOP A POWERFUL V-TAPER

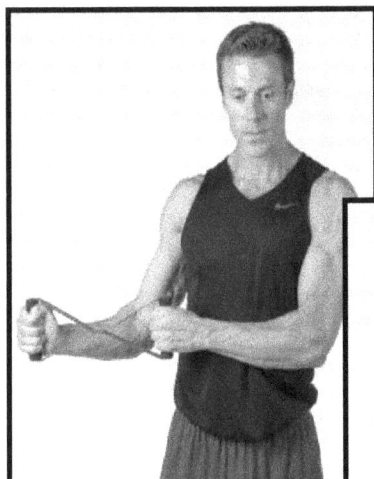

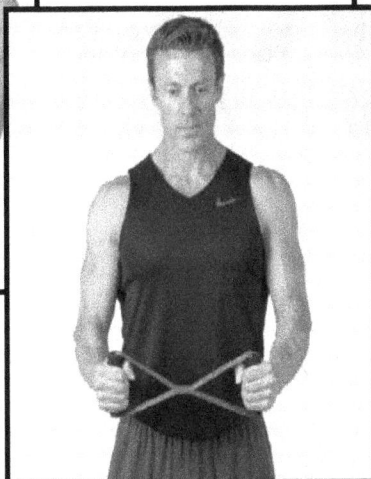

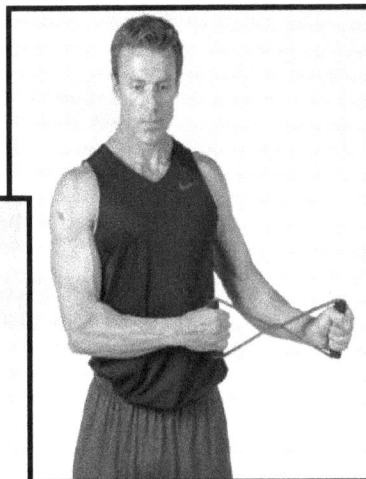

ADD POWER TO THE ROTATOR CUFF MUSCLES

Hold the Iso-Bow as shown. Pull the arms towards the middle of the exercise position, pause for 1 second, then proceed to the opposite side. **RESIST IN A DUAL MANNER**

Chapter 4:

BICEPS
DEVELOP POWERFUL BICEPS

DEVELOP POWERFUL BICEPS

04 DEVELOP POWERFUL BICEPS

The biceps muscle has two heads. A short head, which is on the inside of the arm, and a long head, which is on the outside. This is the part that people see first. The main roll of the biceps is to flex the forearm by bringing the hand towards the shoulder. In order to build powerful complete biceps, you need to learn that the biceps do not work by itself.

The brachialis, which is under the bicep when developed, gives the bicep a larger and fuller appearance. Performing curls place undesirable tension on the tendon near the elbow. In other words, the biceps is placed in a very vulnerable position. Always start all bicep exercises with a slight bend at the start and finish. Always maintain tension on the biceps and not the joint.

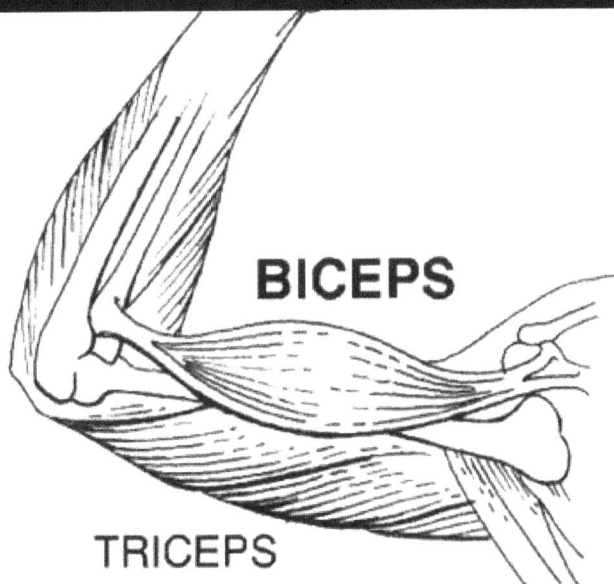

BICEPS

TRICEPS

BICEP EXERCISES

04 DEVELOP POWERFUL BICEPS

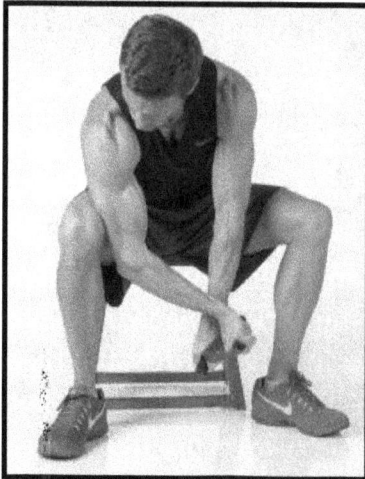

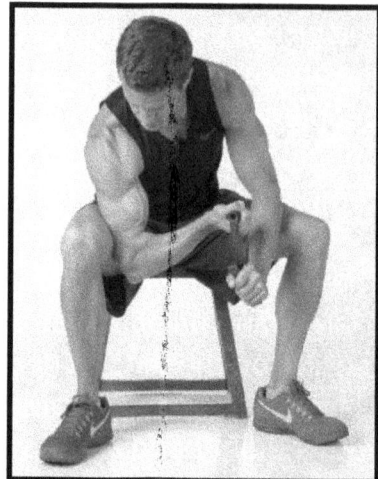

CONCENTRATION CURLS

As pictured, pull the right arm towards the face while resisting with the left hand. Now reverse the exercise by pushing the left arm down and resisting with the right. Complete your reps then switch arms and repeat movement. **DUAL ACTION**

BICEP EXERCISES

04 DEVELOP POWERFUL BICEPS

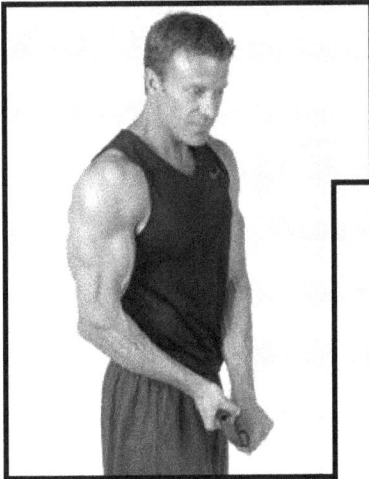

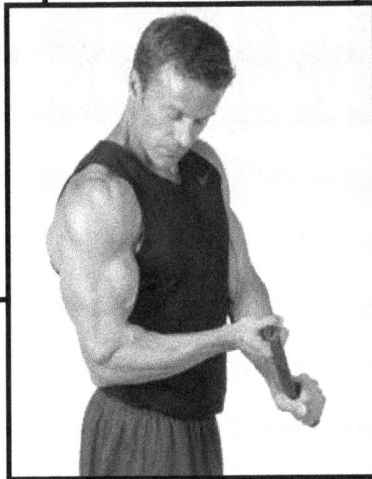

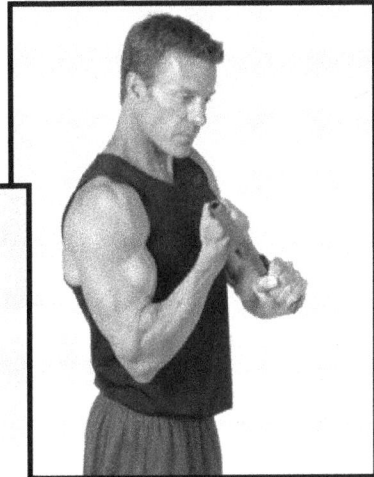

PALM UP CURLS

Pull the right arm upward towards the shoulder while resisting with the left hand. At the shoulder, reverse the exercise by pushing the left arm downwards, resisting with the right.

Chapter 5:

TRICEPS
DEVELOP POWERFUL TRICEPS

DEVELOP POWERFUL TRICEPS

05 DEVELOP POWERFUL TRICEPS

DEVELOP POWERFUL TRICEPS

The triceps has three heads: The lateral head, middle head and the long head. The role of the triceps is to straighten the arm. The triceps work in opposition to the biceps and brachialis muscles. The triceps has three heads this makes it much larger in mass than the biceps and the brachialis.

Unfortunately, most pay attention to the biceps, leaving the triceps under-developed. The lateral head, which is on the outside is what people see first. The triceps are easy to develop and we have made it easy for the trainee to achieve this.

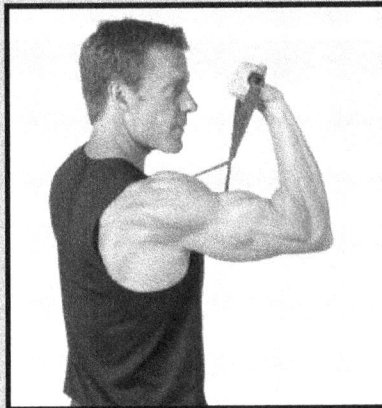

TRICEP EXERCISES

05 DEVELOP POWERFUL TRICEPS

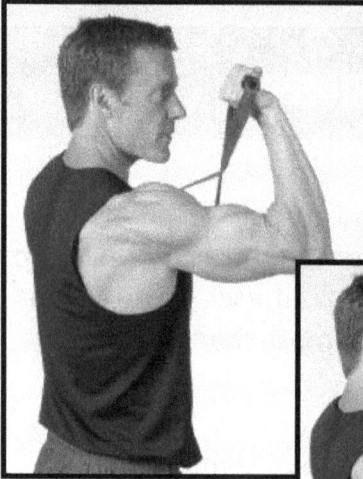

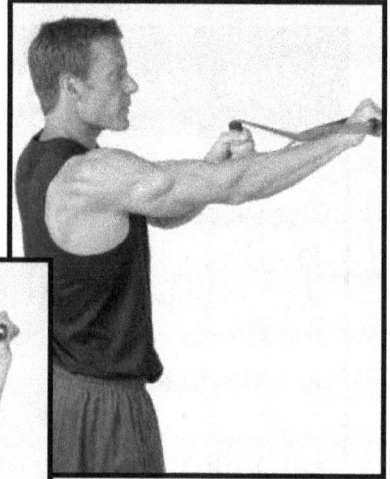

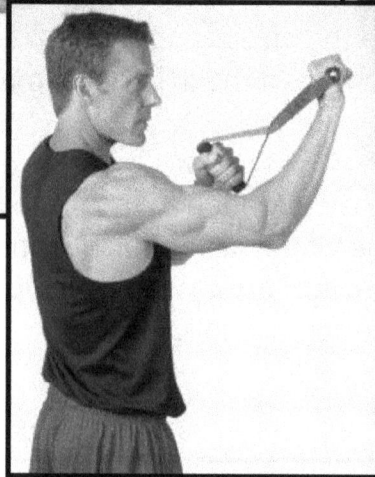

FORWARD EXTENSIONS

As shown above, press the right arm forward while resisting with the left hand. **Do not straighten the elbow.**
RESIST IN A DUAL MANNER

TRICEP EXERCISES

05 DEVELOP POWERFUL TRICEPS

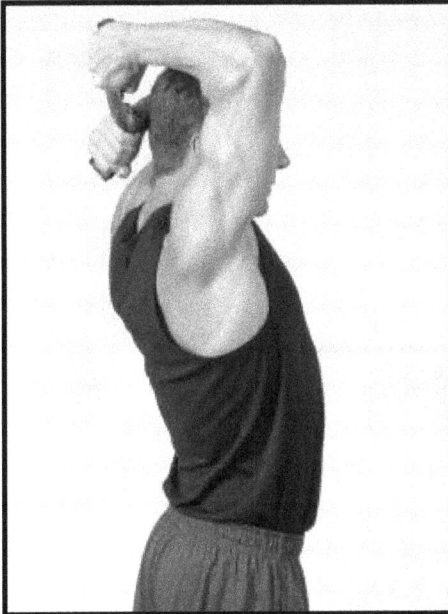

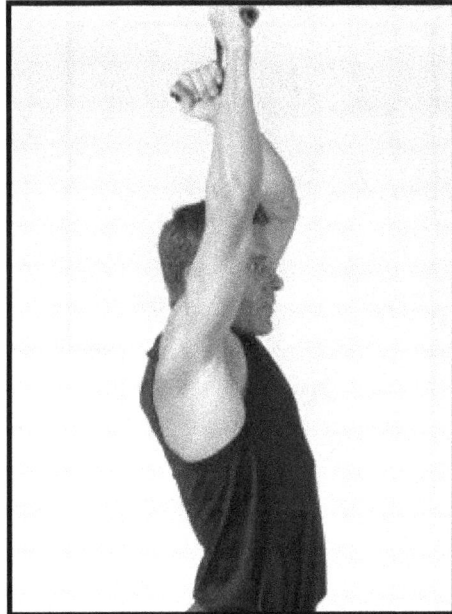

OVERHEAD TRICEP EXTENSIONS

Place arms overhead, press the right arm upwards while resisting with the left arm. Use a light to moderate tension due to the tricep tendons being sensitive at that position. **Do not straighten the elbow. RESIST IN ONE DIRECTION ONLY**

TRICEP EXERCISES

05 DEVELOP POWERFUL TRICEPS

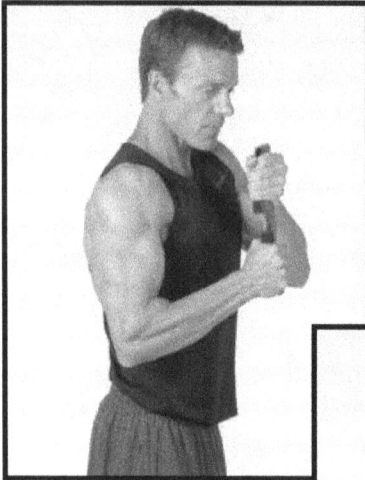

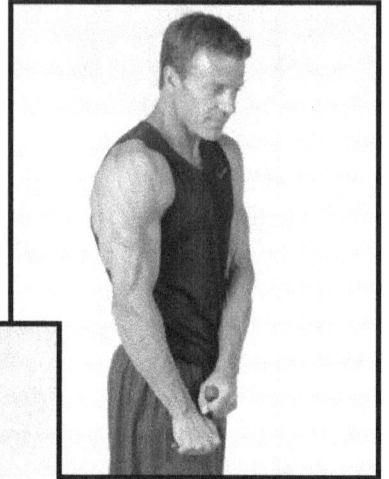

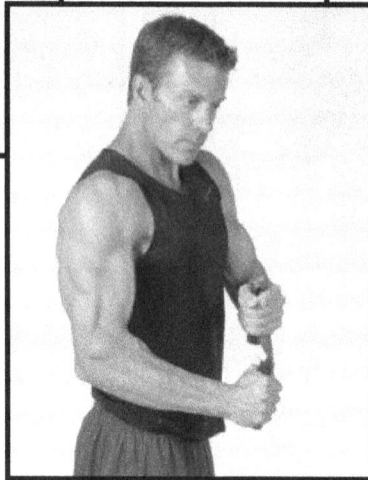

TRICEP PRESSDOWN

As pictured above, press the right hand downwards while resisting with the left arm. Repeat desired reps then switch arms. **RESIST IN ONE DIRECTION ONLY**

DEVELOP RIPPED FOREARMS

05 DEVELOP RIPPED FOREARMS

DEVELOP RIPPED FOREARMS

DEVELOP RIPPED FOREARMS

Forearm muscles are involved in every daily activity, just like the calves and abdominals. We use these muscles all the time, when we drive, write, type, hold a bag and even open a door.

Many of the muscles of the forearm deal with Muscle-multi-use. When you are moving the elbow by lowering and raising the forearm. Moving the wrist up and down by, plus raising and lowering the hand. All self resistance exercises stress the forearms to contract which will increase your grip strength.

FOREARM EXERCISES

05 DEVELOP RIPPED FOREARMS

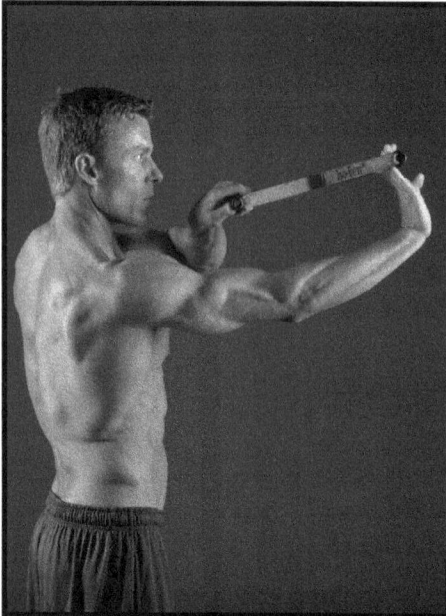

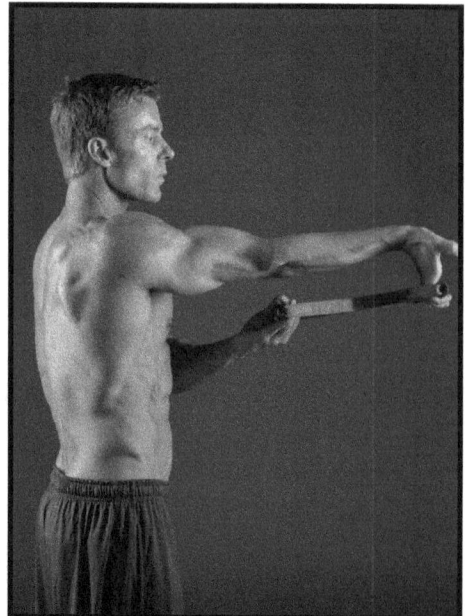

EXERCISE ONE

EXERCISE TWO

HAND/FOREARM EXERCISE

EXERCISE ONE: As pictured press the right hand forward until the fingers are pointed towards your feet. Return to position and repeat. **RESIST IN ONE DIRECTION**

EXERCISE TWO: Same as exercise one but, the hand is placed downwards.

Chapter 6:

THIGHS
DEVELOP POWERFUL THIGHS

DEVELOP POWERFUL TIRELESS THIGHS

06 DEVELOP POWERFUL TIRELESS THIGHS

DEVELOP POWERFUL THIGHS

The thigh muscles are basically made up of four main muscles: the vastus lateral muscle, this is located on the outside of the thighs. The vastus medial muscle, this is located on the inside of the thigh muscles towards the knee.

Better known as the tear drop because of its shape. The recus-femoris, which is located in the center of the muscles, and the vastus intermedius, this muscle is mostly covered by all the other muscles of the thighs. Our program will develop tireless thighs with a power pack punch.

LEG EXERCISES

06 DEVELOP POWERFUL TIRELESS THIGHS

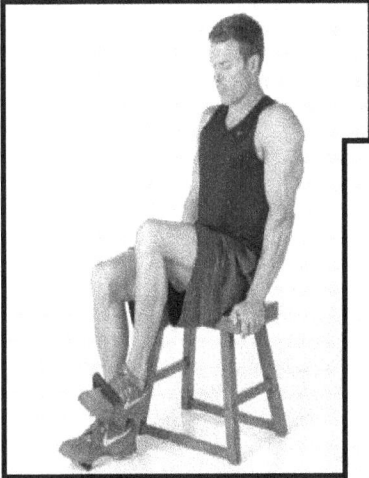

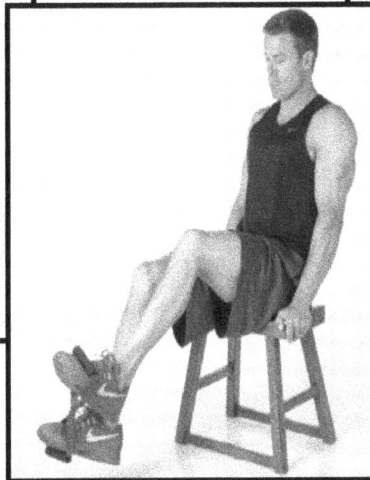

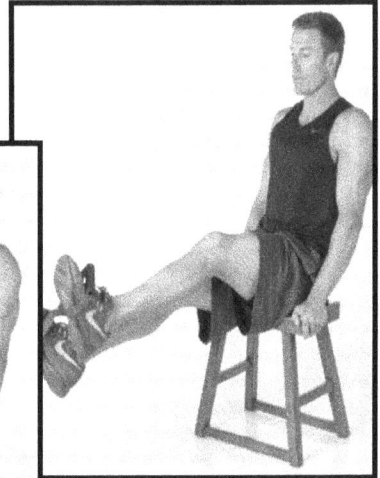

LEG EXTENSIONS

While seated on a chair, box or stool, place the legs as shown in the picture. Now extend the left leg outwards resisting with the right. At the top pause for 2 seconds, then reverse the movement by pulling down with the right while resisting with the left. **DO NOT STRAIGHTEN THE KNEE. RESIST IN A DUAL MANNER**

LEG EXERCISES

06 DEVELOP POWERFUL TIRELESS THIGHS

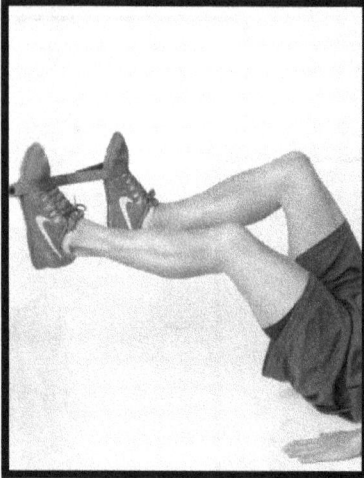

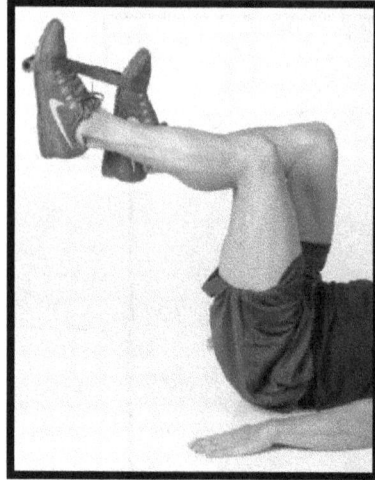

LEG PRESS

As shown, pull the right leg towards the chest, powerfully resisting with the left leg. At the finished position, press the left foot forward resisting with the right. **PERFORM IN A DUAL MANNER**

Chapter 7:

LOWER BACK
DEVELOP POWERFUL LOWER-BACK MUSCLES

DEVELOP POWERFUL LOWER BACK MUSCLES

07 DEVELOP POWERFUL LOWER-BACK MUSCLES

POWERFUL LOWER BACK MUSCLES

Develop Powerful Lower back muscles

The lower back muscles support the lower part of the spine. When these muscles are well developed it builds a brace protecting the spine.

Apart from that the lower back muscles are responsible for bringing the body upright from a leaning forward position. Not only will the lower back be involved, but the glutes and hamstrings come into play.

LOWER BACK EXERCISES

07 DEVELOP POWERFUL LOWER BACK

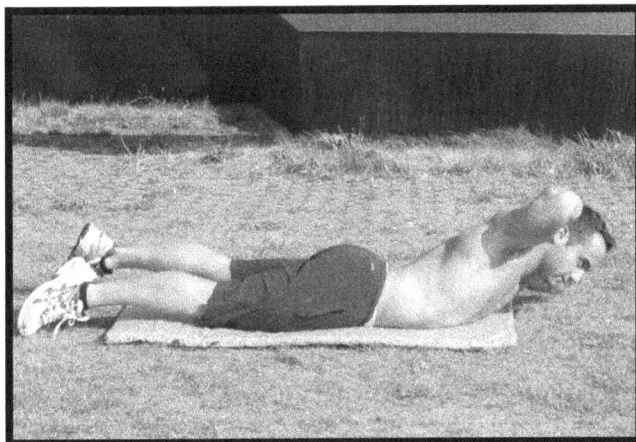

LOWER BACK EXTENSION

As shown above, this is the finished position. Lay flat on the floor and perform this movement by raising the upper body upwards slowly pause for 2 seconds at the top. Then slowly reverse the movement under control.

Chapter 8:

CALVES

DEVELOP SHAPELY CALVES

DEVELOP SHAPELY CALVES

08 DEVELOP SHAPELY CALVES

DEVELOP SHAPELY CALVES

Develop shapely calves

The calves add a finished look to the lower leg with a diamond shape. This muscle has three heads (muscle parts) the soleus, this is under the large lateral head and gives the calves a fully developed look viewed from the side and back.

The lateral and medial heads are on the outside and in the middle of the muscle. The gastrocnemius make up the majority of the calf muscle. However, the longer the gastroc, the larger the potential for enhanced calf muscle development. The stretch component adds strength, shape and muscle development in double quick time.

DEVELOP SHAPELY CALVES

08 DEVELOP SHAPELY CALVES

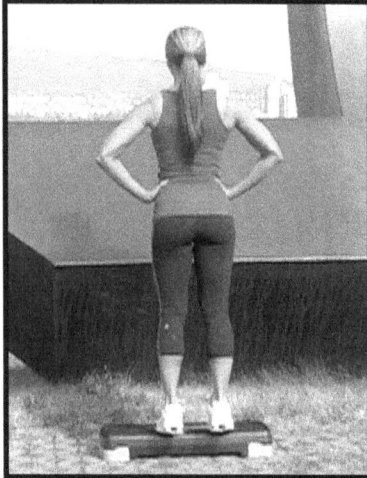

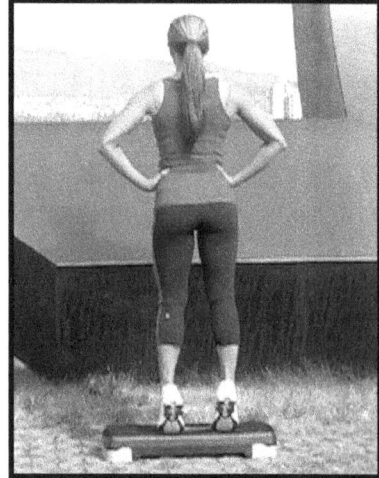

STANDING CALVE RAISES

Position yourself as shown but make sure the calves are well stretched. Start off as shown in the picture start position. Press straight up on the toes then lower. This is as awesome calve stretch exercise. Perform this exercise until the calves are well tired. This stimulates the entire calve.

Chapter 9:

ABDOMINALS
DEVELOP RIPPED ABS

DEVELOP RIPPED ABS

09 DEVELOP RIPPED ABS

The abdominal muscles are very important and reveal that the trainee has a lean physique. Plus, the role of the abdominal muscles is to protect the spine. A lean chiseled set of abdominal muscles shows the opposite sex that the owner has a sign of virility.

Once these muscles are well developed this keeps the waist line and belly flat. There are various muscle structures that complete the overall look, the entire length of the abdominal wall, plus the internal and external obliques.

The lower sections of the abdominal muscles play the largest role in protecting the spine and storing belly fat. This is the easiest place for body-fat to accumulate. Which makes training with self resistance the ideal exercise to attack those muscle fibers to the maximum.

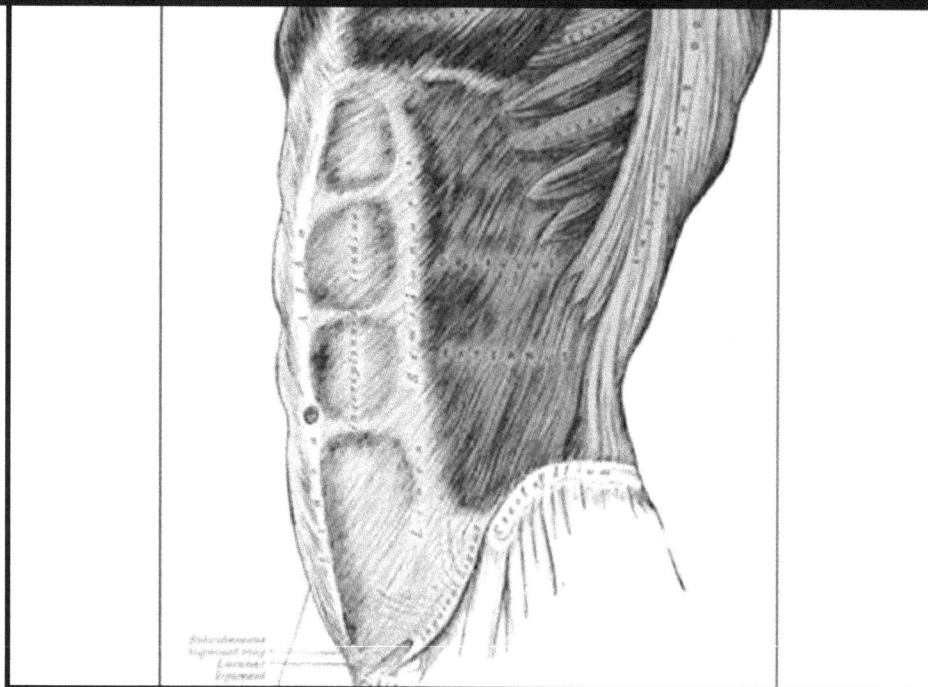

DEVELOP RIPPED ABS

09 DEVELOP RIPPED ABS

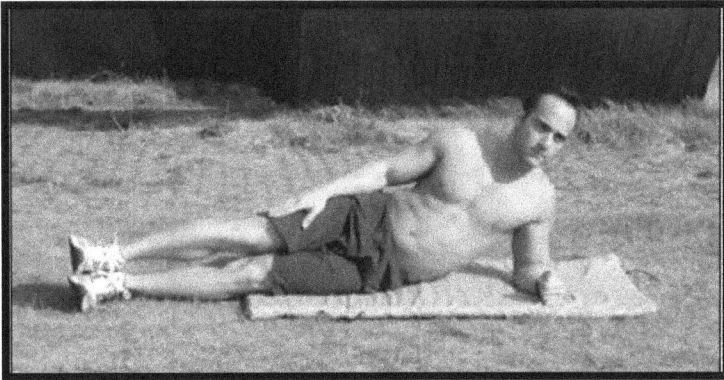

DEVELOP RIPPED ABDOMINALS

As noted in the introduction the abdominal wall includes four muscles:
Let's cover the entire length from the chest to pubis is called the rectus
abdominis, people say abs for short. The abdominal wall should be worked
in three angles of flexion. The lower sections of the abdominal muscles.
The upper sections of the abdominal wall, and the obliques. Which are
rotator muscles.

DEVELOP RIPPED ABS

09 DEVELOP RIPPED ABS

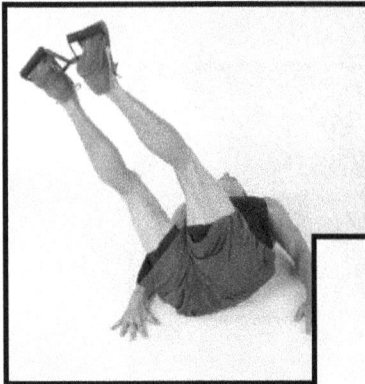

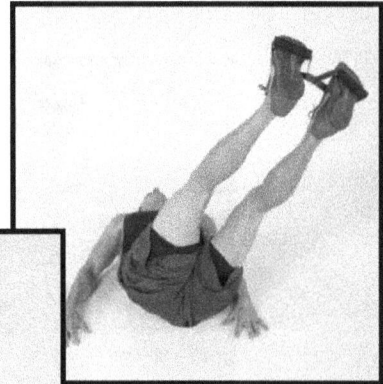

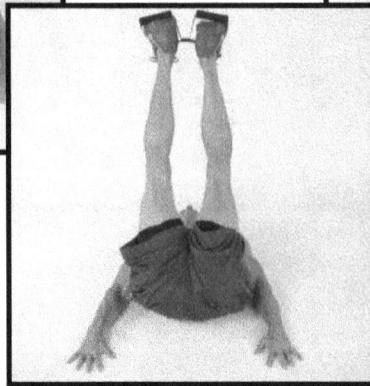

SIDE TO SIDE LATERAL RAISES

Normally people say I want to get rid of my love handles.
This abdominal exercise really isolates the oblique muscles.
These muscles support the spine by making the abdominal wall
more rigid. Start off as shown, spread the Iso-Bow apart maintaining the tension, Then lower the legs side to side.

DEVELOP RIPPED ABS

09 DEVELOP RIPPED ABS

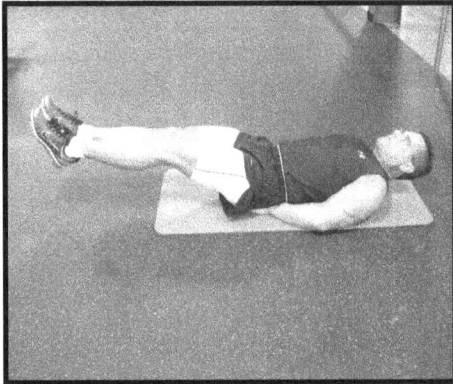

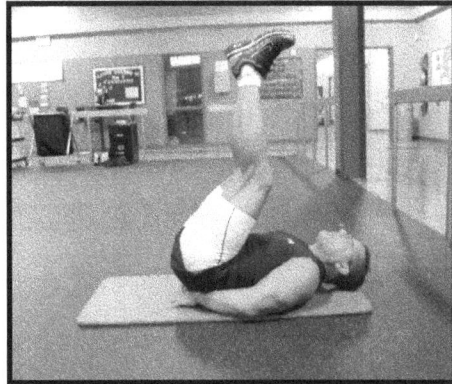

REVERSE CRUNCHES

As shown above, place your hands under your butt slowly raise the legs upwards towards the chest or stomach. Pause for a 1 second count then slowly reverse the movement. This exercise stimulates the entire abdominal wall.

DEVELOP RIPPED ABS

09 DEVELOP RIPPED ABS

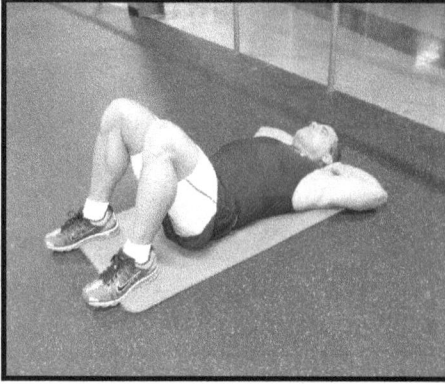

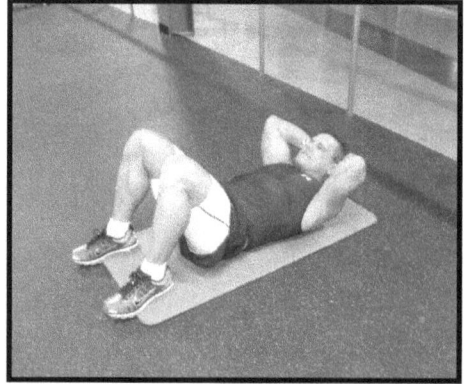

ABDOMINAL CRUNCHES

Lay on your back. Place the hands at your ear, tilt your head back, focus on the ceiling and crunch upward as shown.
DO NOT PULL ON THE HEAD.

Chapter 10:

POWER PUMP

PHASE ONE

PROGRAM

**REP SPEED ON THIS PHASE 3 SECONDS CONTRACTED
6 SECONDS RELEASE.
ALL PHASES ARE PERFORMED FOR 2 WEEKS IN CIRCUIT STYLE
DO NOT SKIP PHASES**

POWER PUMP PROGRAM PHASE ONE

10 PHASE ONE

MONDAY, WEDNESDAY, FRIDAY

Perform 5 reps each exercise until all exercises are completed. On the 5th rep perform a 10 second Isometric contraction at the mid-point of the exercise stroke. Example...middle position on the bicep curl.
Perform 2 circuits.

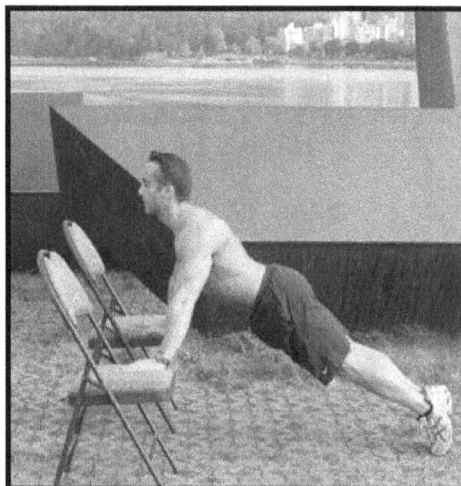

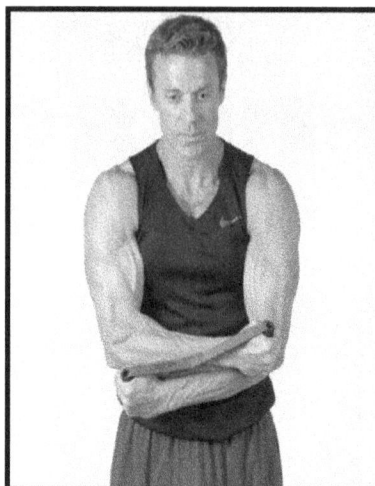

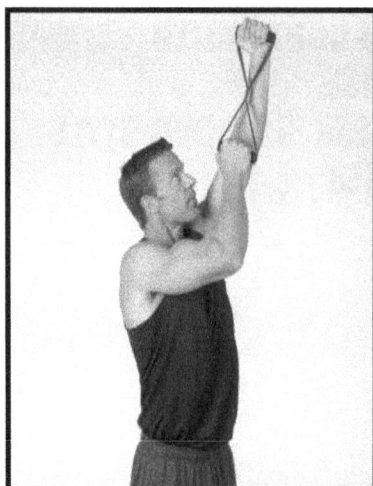

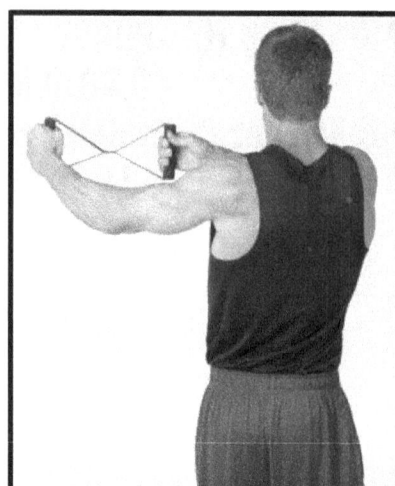

POWER PUMP PROGRAM PHASE ONE

10 PHASE ONE

MONDAY, WEDNESDAY, FRIDAY
Routine continued.........

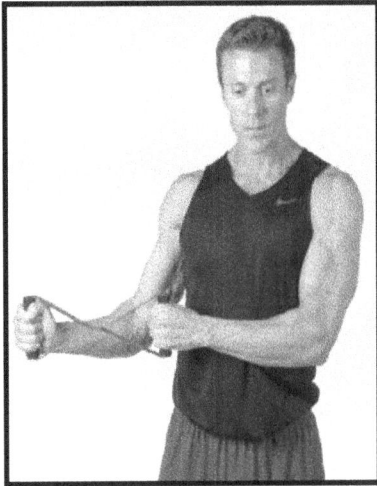

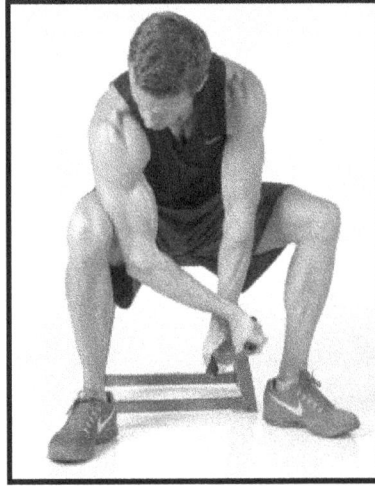

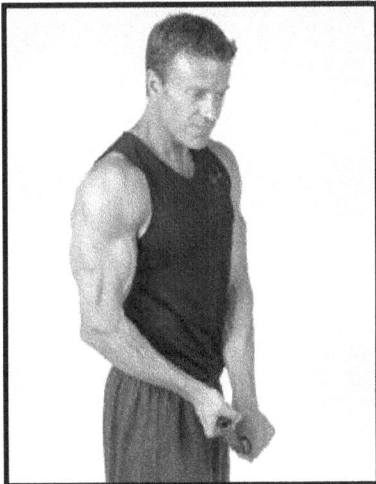

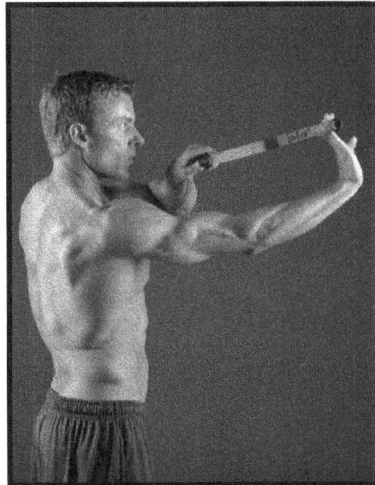

POWER PUMP PROGRAM PHASE ONE

10 PHASE ONE

MONDAY, WEDNESDAY, FRIDAY
Routine continued...........

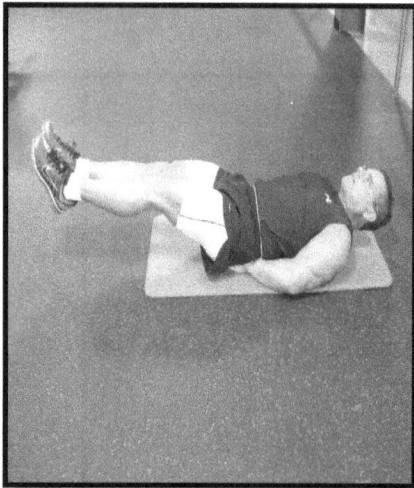

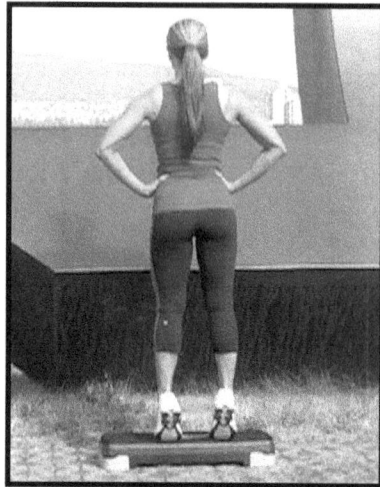

PHASE ONE MON, WED, FRI

POWER PUMP PROGRAM PHASE ONE

10 PHASE ONE

TUESDAY, THURSDAY, SATURDAY

Perform 5 reps each exercise until all exercises are completed. On the 5th rep perform a 10 second Isometric contraction at the contracted position of the exercise stroke. Example...Top position on the lateral raise, top position on the bicep curl. **Perform 2 circuits.**

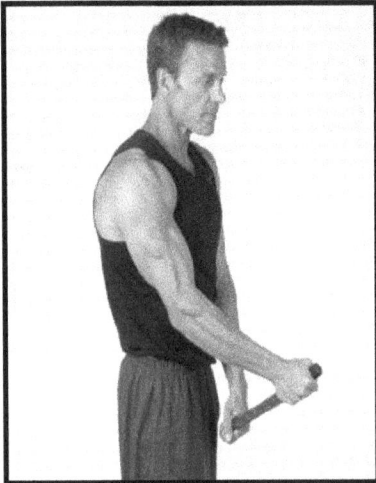

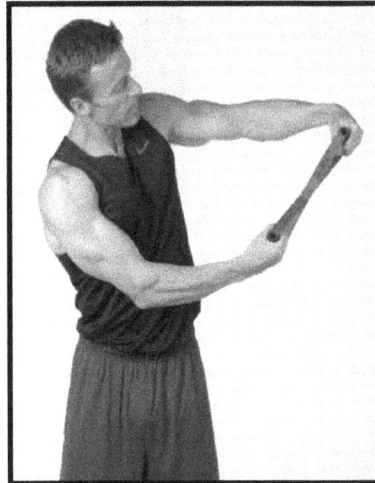

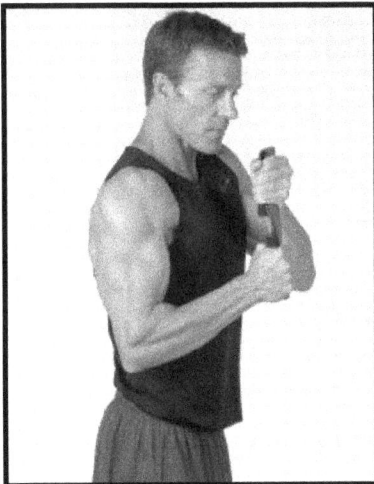

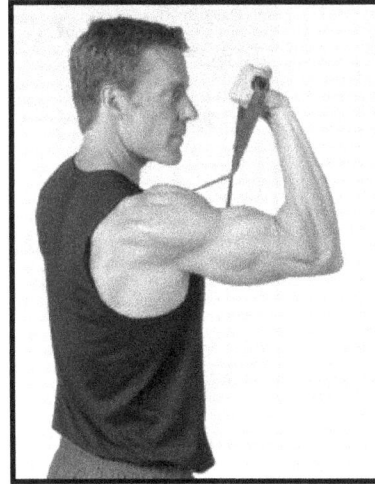

POWER PUMP PROGRAM PHASE ONE

10 PHASE ONE

TUESDAY, THURSDAY, SATURDAY
Continued routine..........

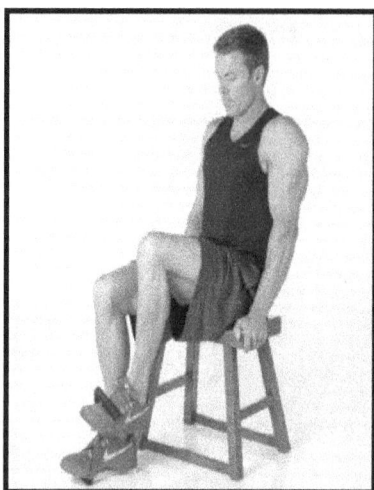

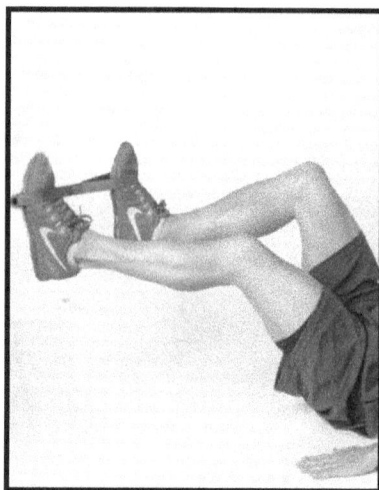

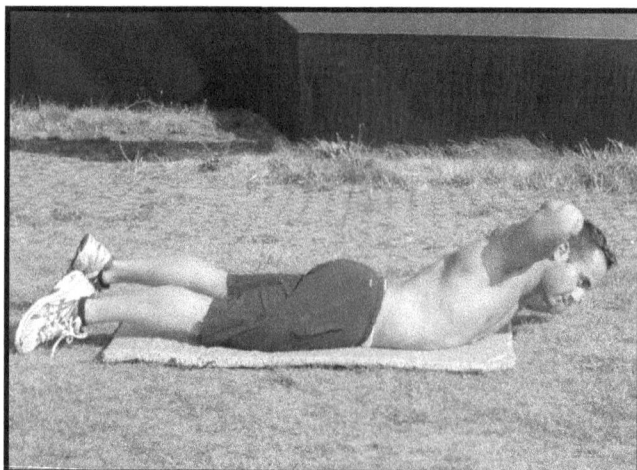

POWER PUMP PROGRAM PHASE ONE

10 PHASE ONE

TUESDAY, THURSDAY, SATURDAY
Continued routine........

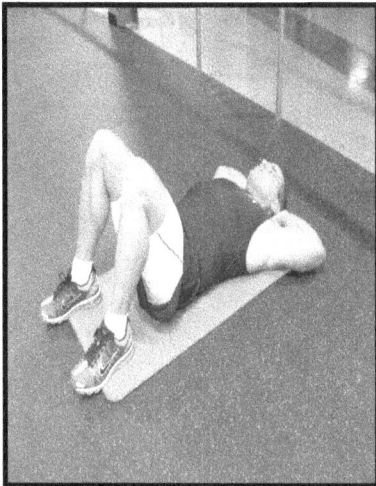

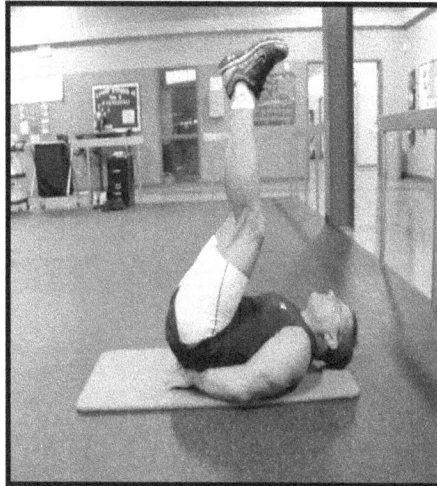

PHASE ONE TUES, THURS, SAT.

POWER PUMP PROGRAM PHASE TWO

11 PHASE TWO

MONDAY, WEDNESDAY, FRIDAY

Perform 7 reps each exercise until all exercises are completed. On the 7th rep perform a 5 second Isometric contraction at the middle position of the exercise stroke. Example...Middle position on the lateral raise, middle position on the bicep curl. **Perform 2 circuits.**

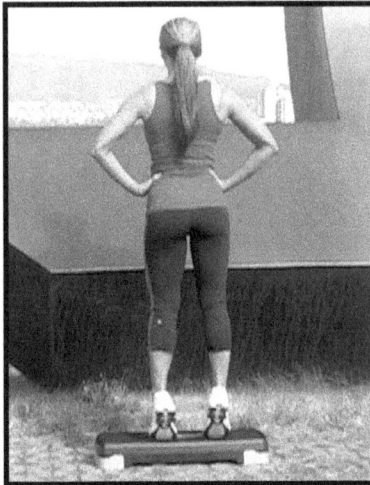

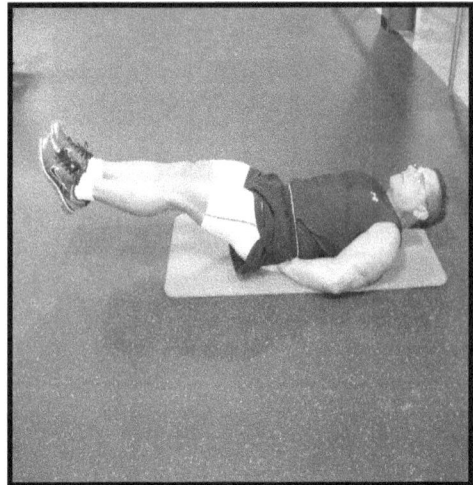

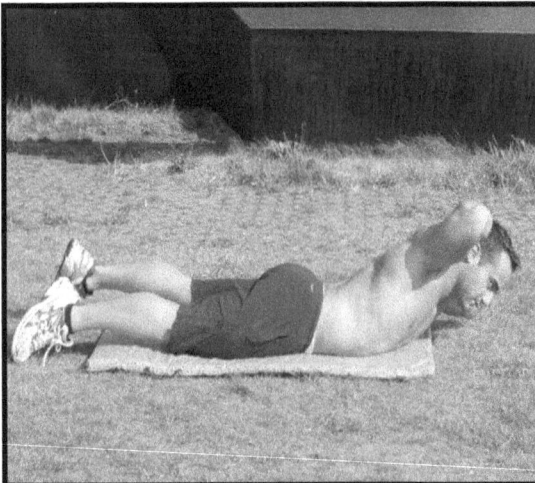

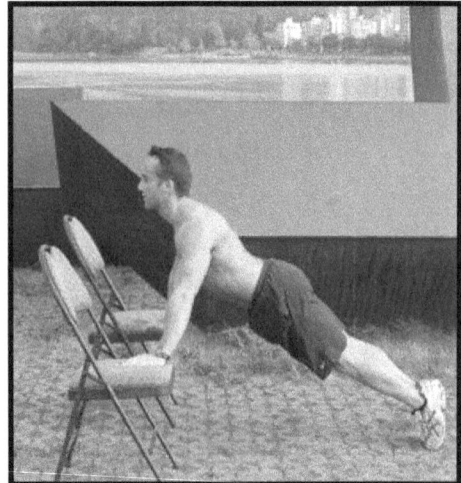

POWER PUMP PROGRAM PHASE TWO

11 PHASE TWO

MONDAY, WEDNESDAY, FRIDAY
ROUTINE CONTINUED........

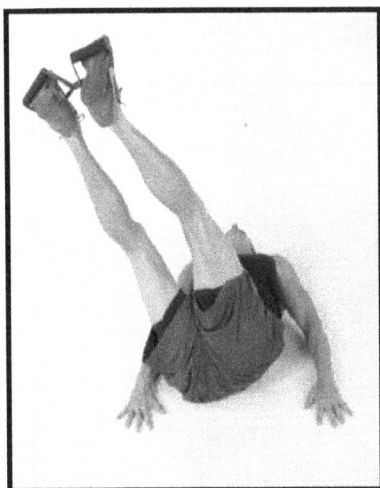

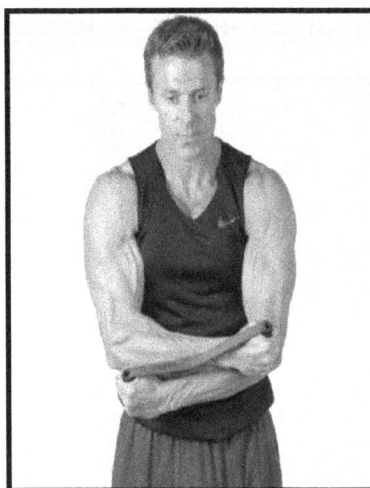

PHASE TWO   MON, WED, FRI.

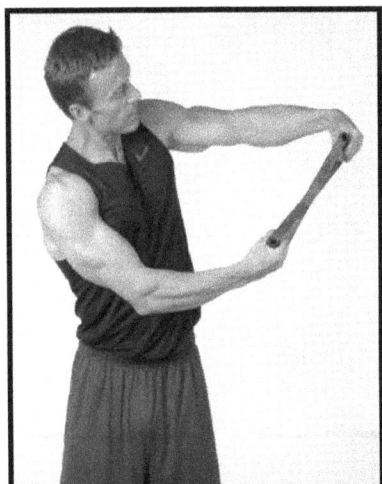

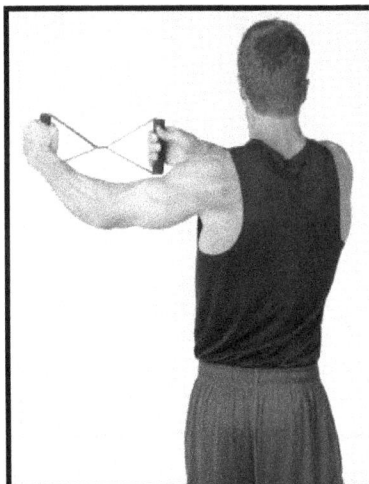

POWER PUMP PROGRAM PHASE TWO

11 PHASE TWO

TUESDAY, THURSDAY, SATURDAY

Perform 7 reps each exercise until all exercises are completed. On the 7th rep perform a 5 second Isometric contraction at the middle position of the exercise stroke. Example...Middle position on the lateral raise, middle position on the bicep curl. **Perform 2 circuits.**

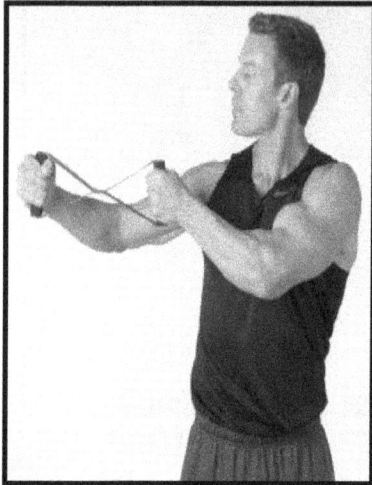

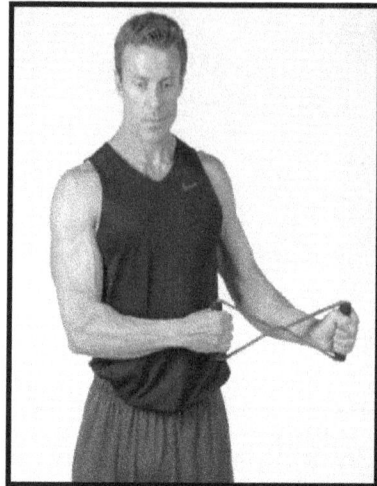

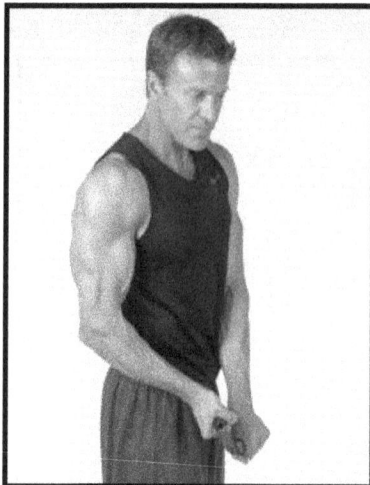

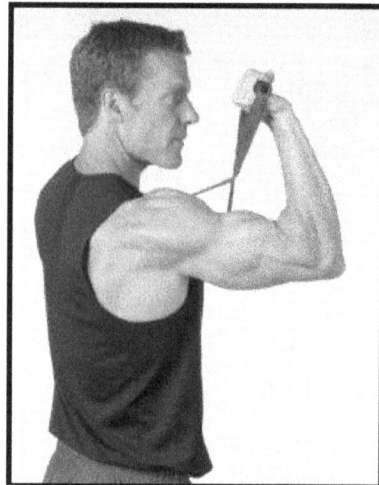

POWER PUMP PROGRAM PHASE TWO

11 PHASE TWO

TUESDAY, THURSDAY, SATURDAY

ROUTINE CONTINUED..........

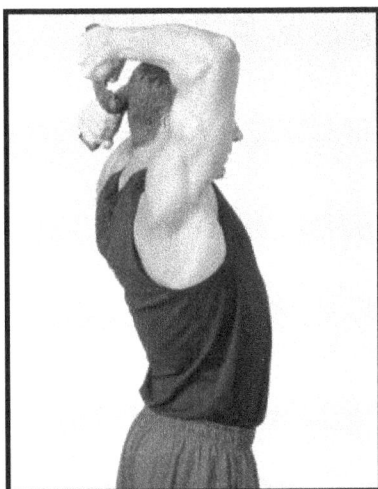

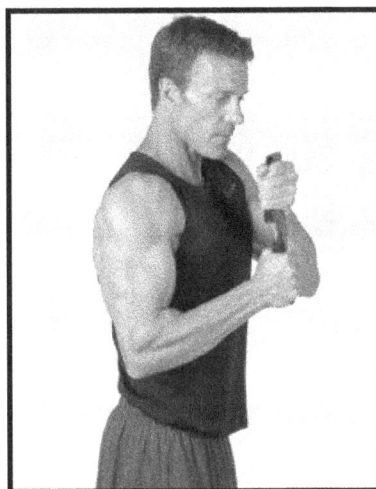

PHASE TWO   TUES, THURS, SAT.

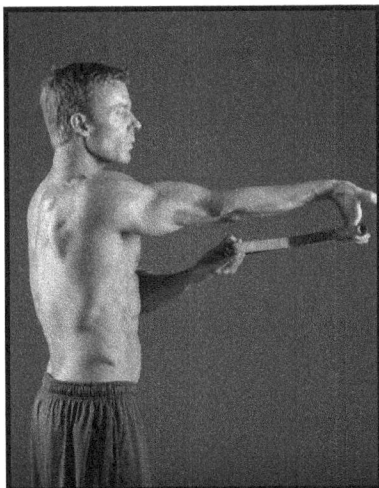

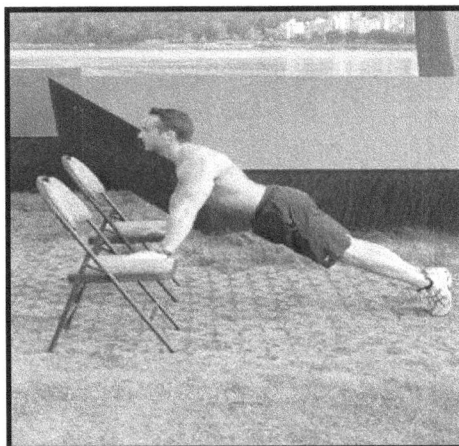

Chapter 12:

MUSCLE BLAST
FIBER MAX POINT

WEEK ONE: 20 REPS PER EXERCISE
WEEK TWO: 15 REPS PER EXERCISE
WEEK THREE: 10 REPS PER EXERCISE

**ON RESISTANCE EXERCISES PERFORM A 10 SECOND
ISOMETRIC CONTRACTION BEFORE REPS.
REP SPEED 3 SECONDS CONTRACTED, 3 SECONDS RELEASE**

PERFORM PROGRAM 3 WEEKS

FIBER MAX POINT

12 FIBER MAX POINT

HOW TO PERFORM THIS ROUTINE:
WEEK ONE: 20 Reps per exercise
WEEK TWO: 15 Reps per exercise
WEEK THREE: 10 Reps per exercise
PERFORM 2 CIRCUITS

DAY ONE

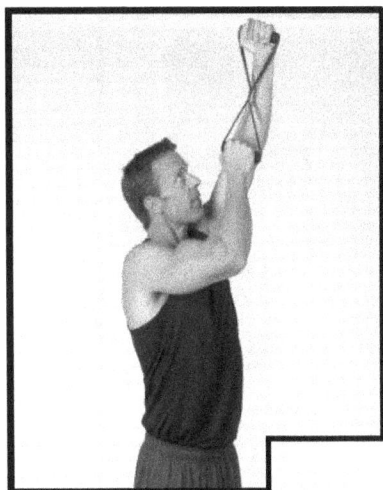
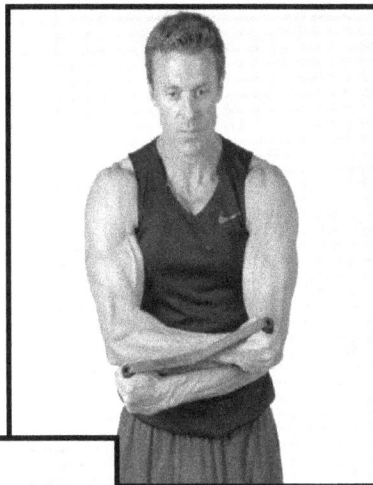
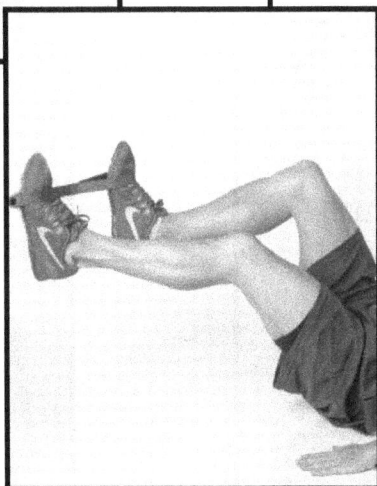

FIBER MAX POINT

12 FIBER MAX POINT

HOW TO PERFORM THIS ROUTINE:
WEEK ONE: 20 Reps per exercise
WEEK TWO: 15 Reps per exercise
WEEK THREE: 10 Reps per exercise
PERFORM 2 CIRCUITS

DAY ONE continued.........

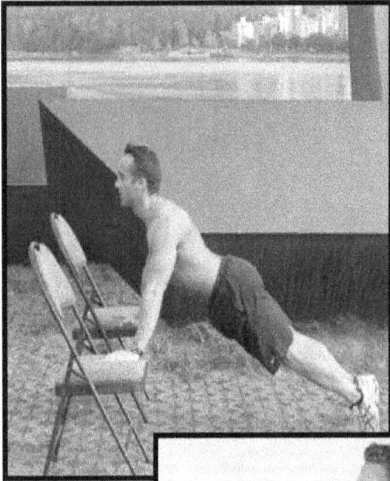
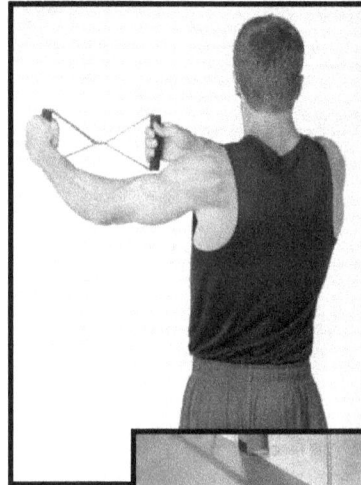
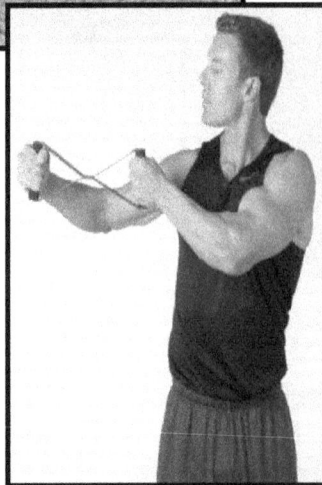
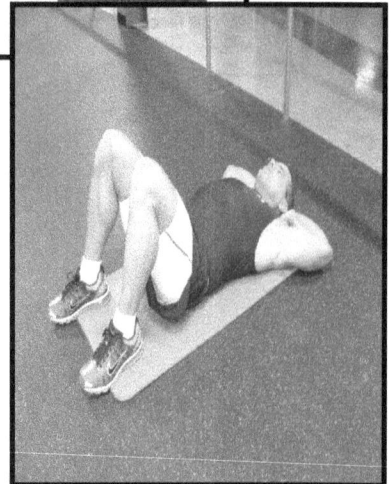

FIBER MAX POINT

12 FIBER MAX POINT

HOW TO PERFORM THIS ROUTINE:
WEEK ONE: 20 Reps per exercise
WEEK TWO: 15 Reps per exercise
WEEK THREE: 10 Reps per exercise
PERFORM 2 CIRCUITS

DAY TWO

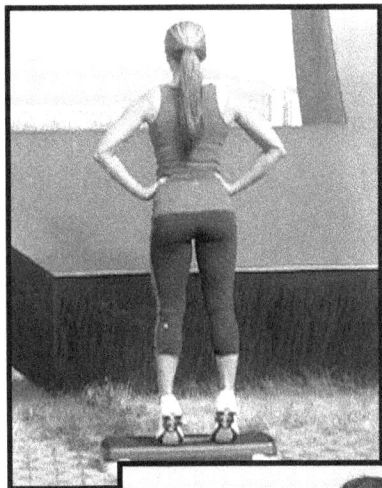

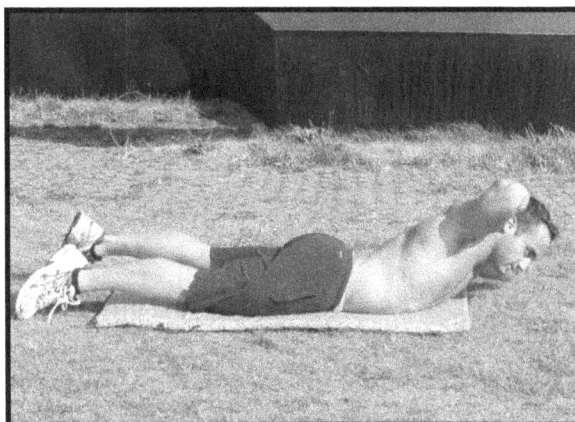

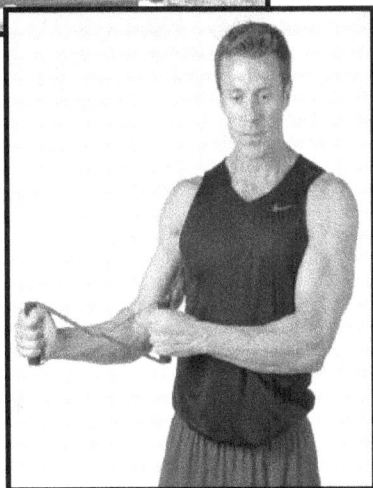

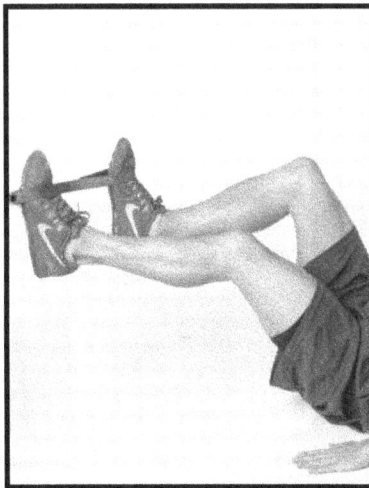

FIBER MAX POINT

12 FIBER MAX POINT

HOW TO PERFORM THIS ROUTINE:
WEEK ONE: 20 Reps per exercise
WEEK TWO: 15 Reps per exercise
WEEK THREE: 10 Reps per exercise
PERFORM 2 CIRCUITS

DAY TWO continued............

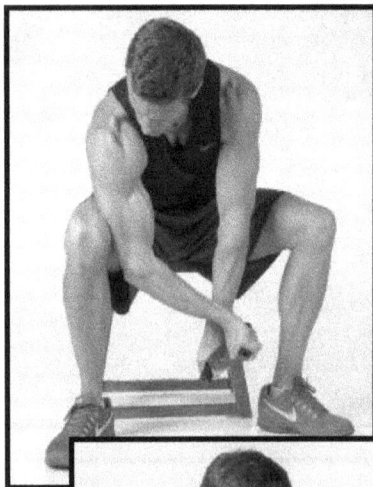

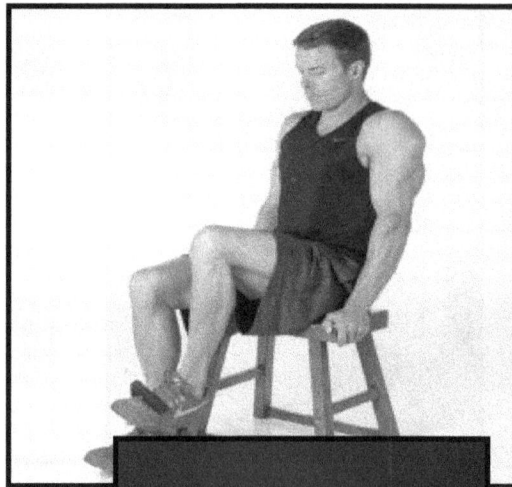

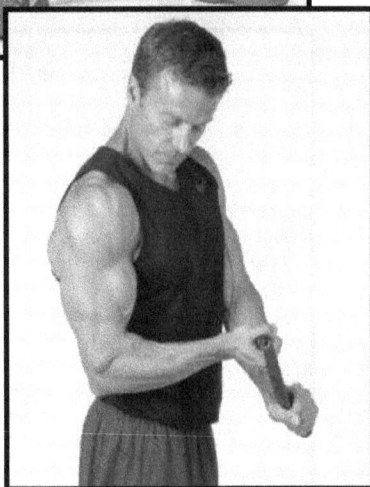

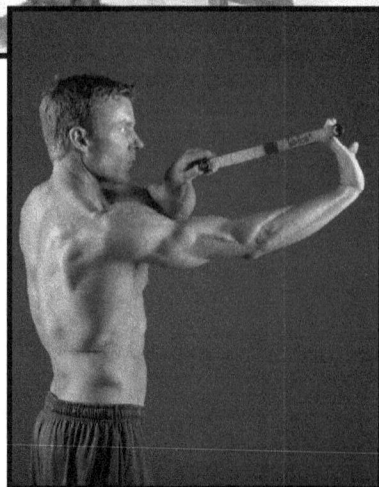

FIBER MAX POINT

12 FIBER MAX POINT

HOW TO PERFORM THIS ROUTINE:
WEEK ONE: 20 Reps per exercise
WEEK TWO: 15 Reps per exercise
WEEK THREE: 10 Reps per exercise
PERFORM 2 CIRCUITS

DAY THREE

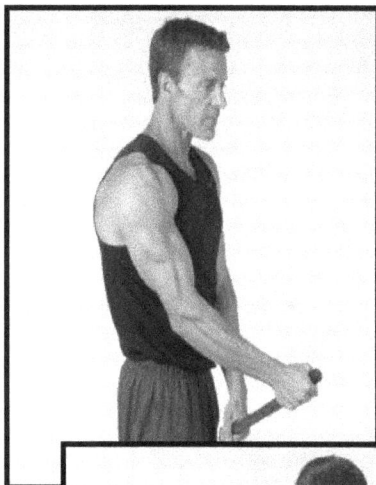
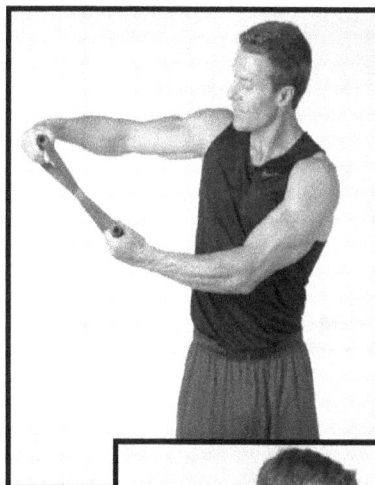
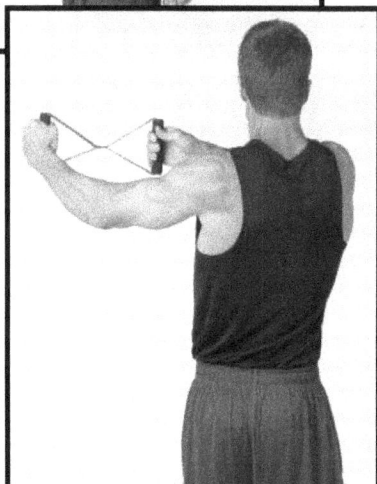
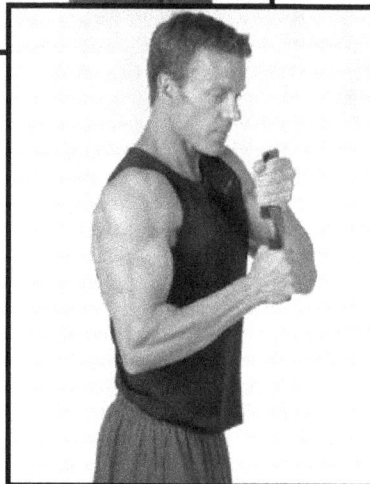

FIBER MAX POINT

12 FIBER MAX POINT

HOW TO PERFORM THIS ROUTINE:
WEEK ONE: 20 Reps per exercise
WEEK TWO: 15 Reps per exercise
WEEK THREE: 10 Reps per exercise
PERFORM 2 CIRCUITS

DAY THREE continued......

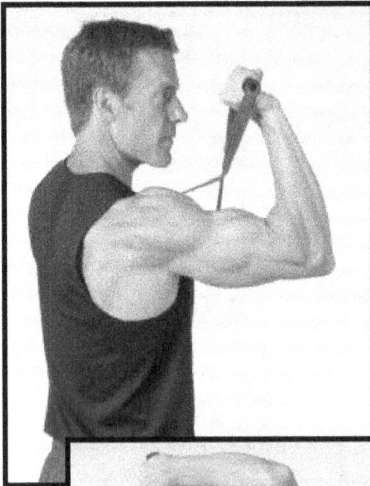

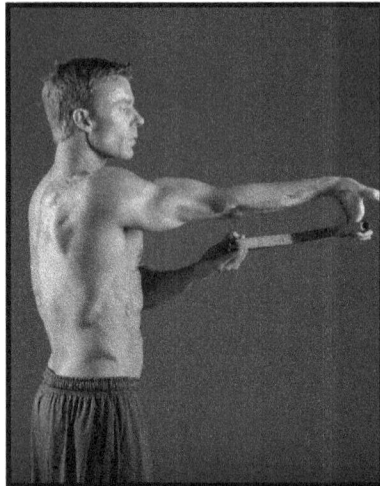

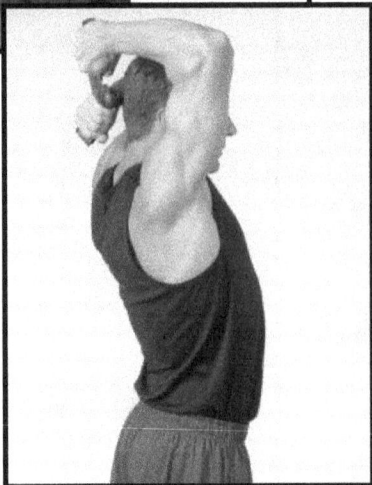

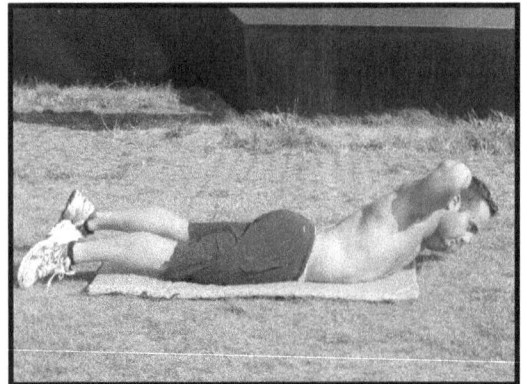

FIBER MAX POINT

12 FIBER MAX POINT

HOW TO PERFORM THIS ROUTINE:
WEEK ONE: 20 Reps per exercise
WEEK TWO: 15 Reps per exercise
WEEK THREE: 10 Reps per exercise
PERFORM 2 CIRCUITS

DAY THREE continued......

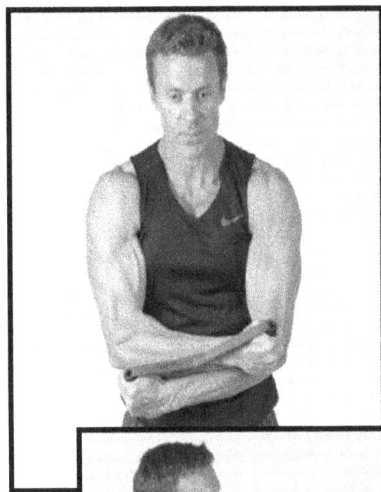

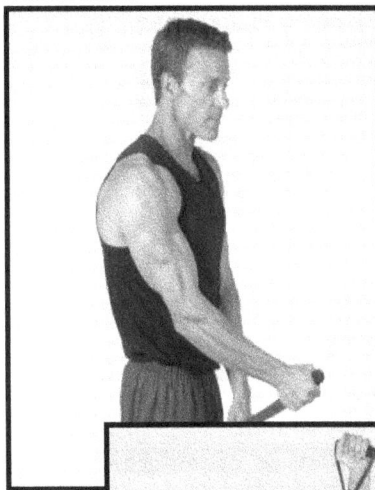

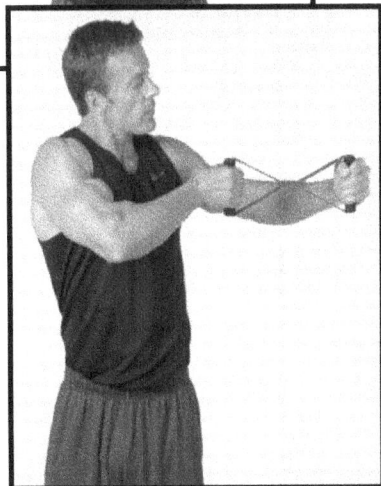

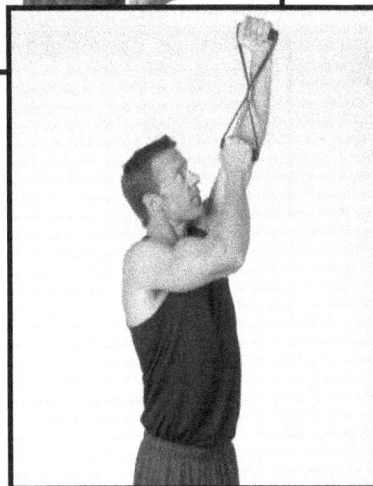

FIBER MAX POINT

12 FIBER MAX POINT

HOW TO PERFORM THIS ROUTINE:
WEEK ONE: 20 Reps per exercise
WEEK TWO: 15 Reps per exercise
WEEK THREE: 10 Reps per exercise
PERFORM 2 CIRCUITS

DAY FOUR

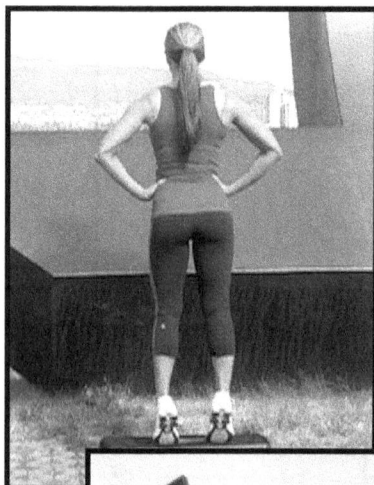
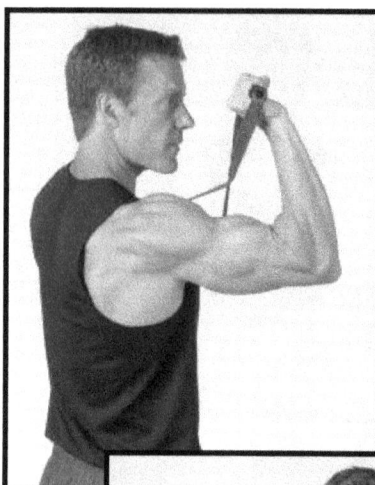
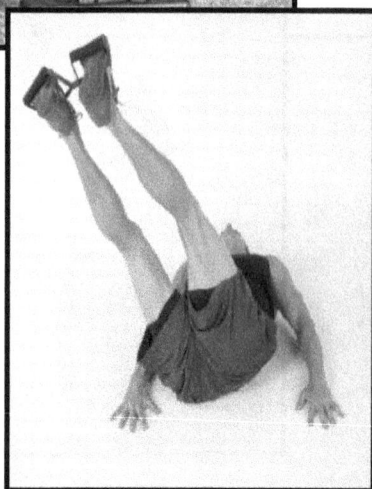
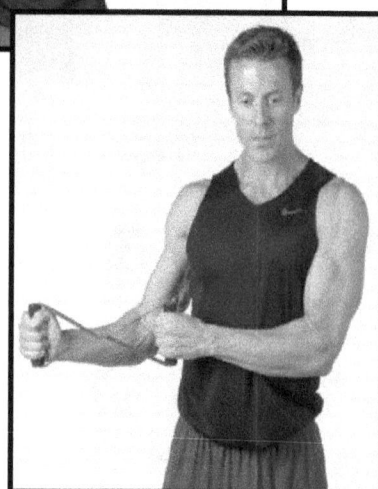

FIBER MAX POINT

12 FIBER MAX POINT

HOW TO PERFORM THIS ROUTINE:
WEEK ONE: 20 Reps per exercise
WEEK TWO: 15 Reps per exercise
WEEK THREE: 10 Reps per exercise
PERFORM 2 CIRCUITS

DAY FOUR continued......

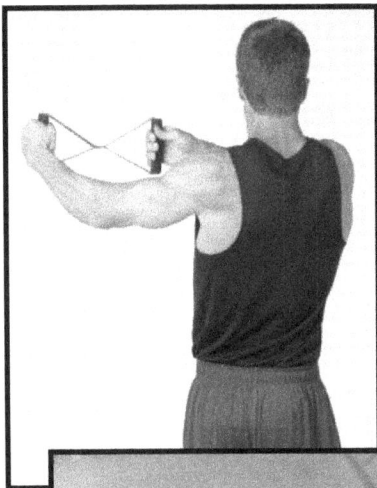

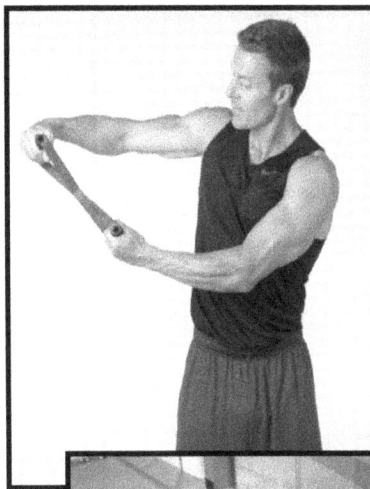

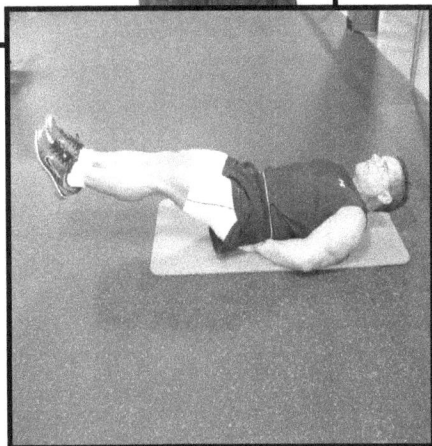

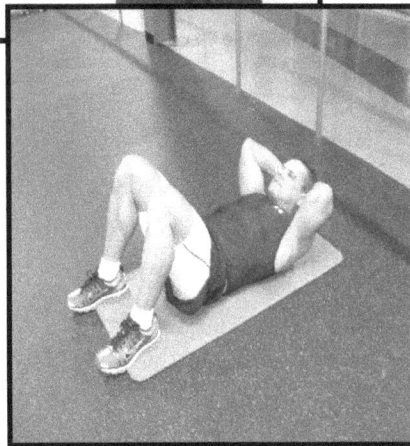

FIBER MAX POINT

12 FIBER MAX POINT

HOW TO PERFORM THIS ROUTINE:
WEEK ONE: 20 Reps per exercise
WEEK TWO: 15 Reps per exercise
WEEK THREE: 10 Reps per exercise
PERFORM 2 CIRCUITS

DAY FIVE

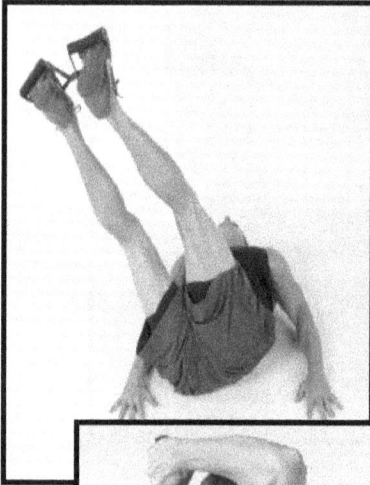

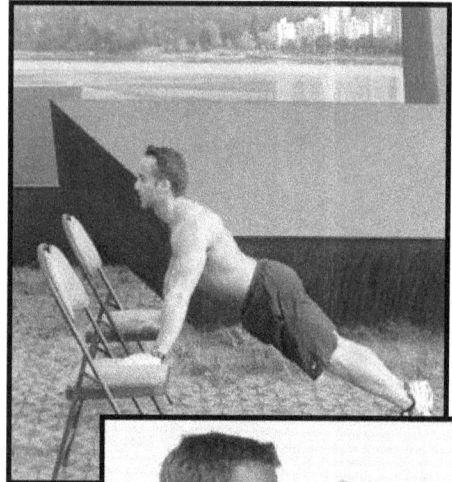

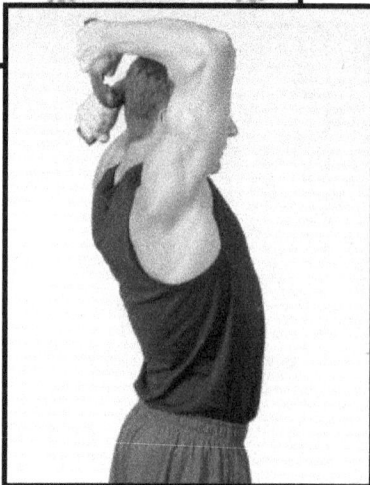

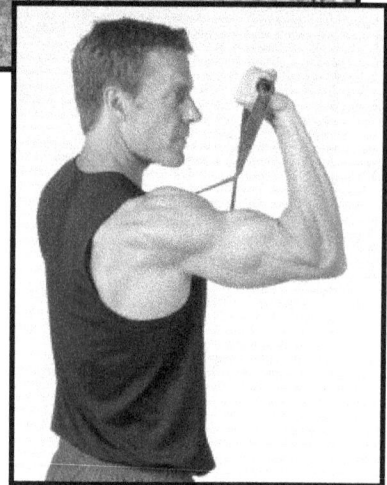

FIBER MAX POINT

12 FIBER MAX POINT

HOW TO PERFORM THIS ROUTINE:
WEEK ONE: 20 Reps per exercise
WEEK TWO: 15 Reps per exercise
WEEK THREE: 10 Reps per exercise
PERFORM 2 CIRCUITS

DAY FIVE continued.....

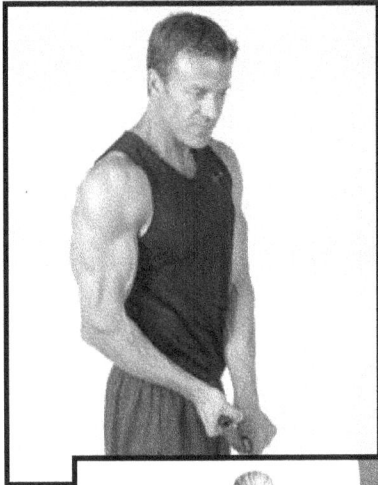

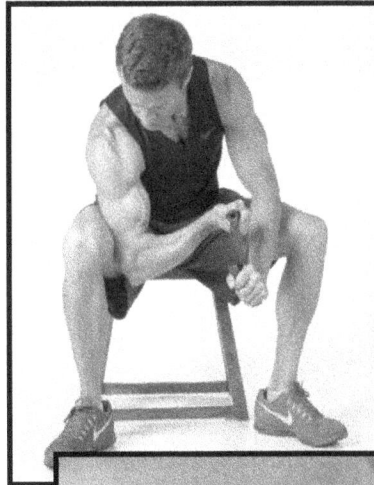

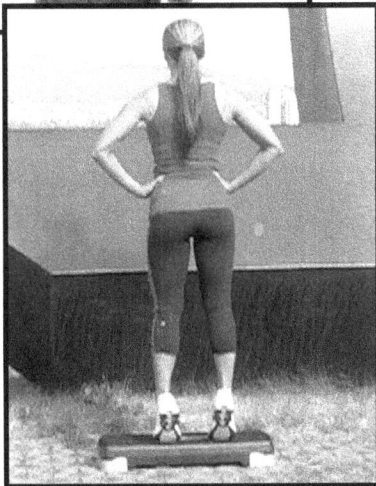

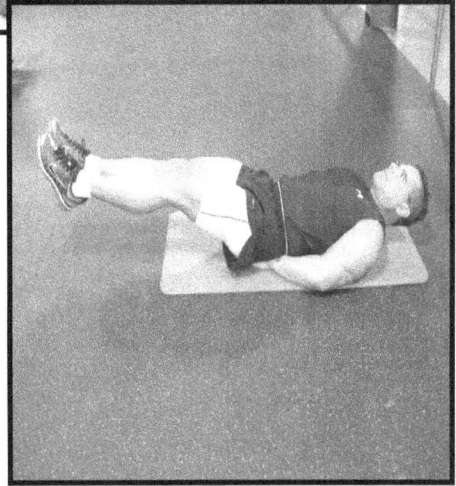

Chapter 13:

THE POWER PUMP
MAX PUMP X1
PROGRAM
PHASE ONE

REP SPEED 3 SECONDS CONTRACTED, 3 SECONDS RELEASE

MAX PUMP X1 PROGRAM

13 PHASE ONE

HOW TO PERFORM THIS ROUTINE:
WEEK ONE: 18 Reps per exercise
WEEK TWO: 25 Reps per exercise
WEEK THREE: 5-6 Reps per exercise
PERFORM A ISOMETRIC CONTRACTION AT THE HALF WAY MARK FOR 5-7 SECONDS
AT THE END OF THE WORK SET. PERFORM 1-2 CIRCUITS

DAY ONE

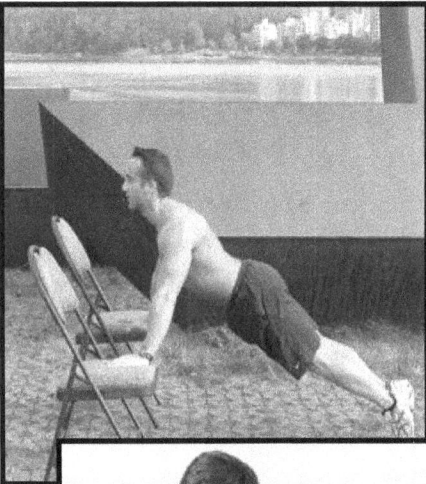
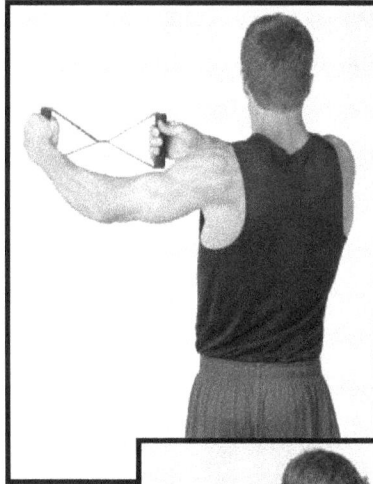
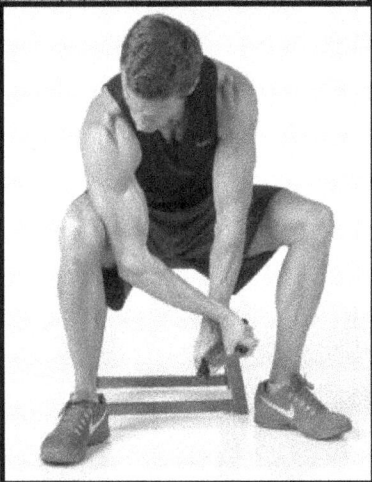
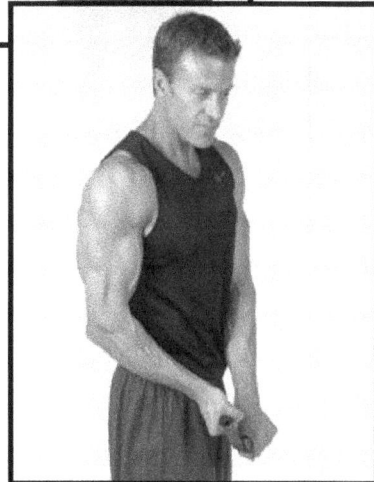

MAX PUMP X1 PROGRAM

13 PHASE ONE

HOW TO PERFORM THIS ROUTINE:
WEEK ONE: 18 Reps per exercise
WEEK TWO: 25 Reps per exercise
WEEK THREE: 5-6 Reps per exercise
PERFORM A ISOMETRIC CONTRACTION AT THE HALF WAY MARK FOR 5-7 SECONDS AT THE END OF THE WORK SET. PERFORM 1-2 CIRCUITS

DAY ONE continued............

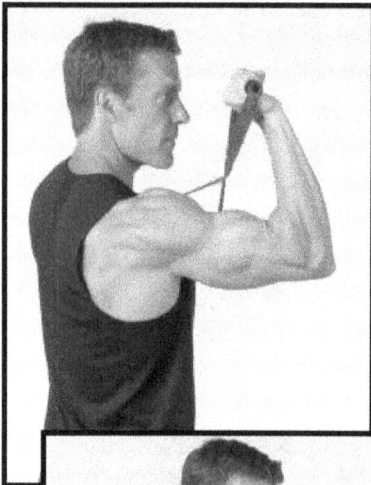
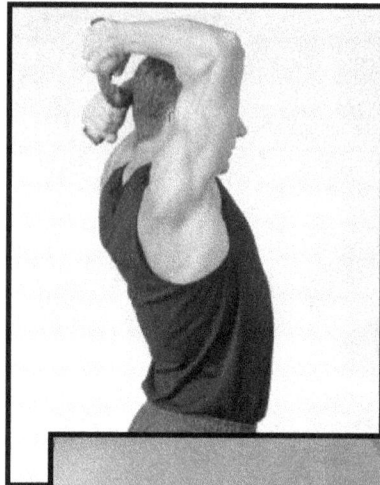
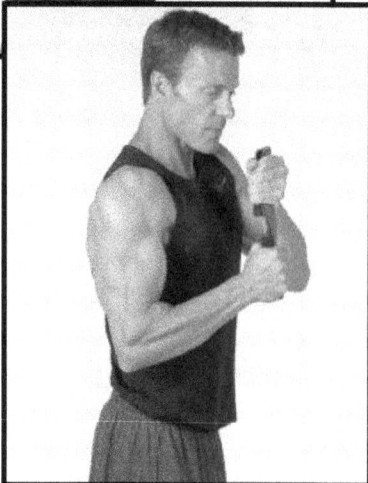
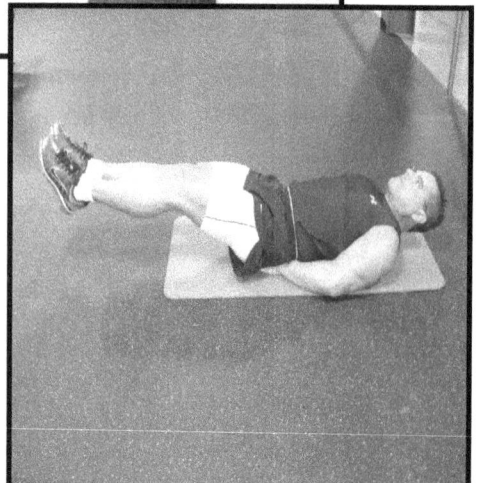

MAX PUMP X1 PROGRAM

13 PHASE ONE

HOW TO PERFORM THIS ROUTINE:
WEEK ONE: 18 Reps per exercise
WEEK TWO: 25 Reps per exercise
WEEK THREE: 5-6 Reps per exercise
**PERFORM A ISOMETRIC CONTRACTION AT THE HALF WAY MARK FOR 5-7 SECONDS
AT THE END OF THE WORK SET. PERFORM 1-2 CIRCUITS**

DAY TWO

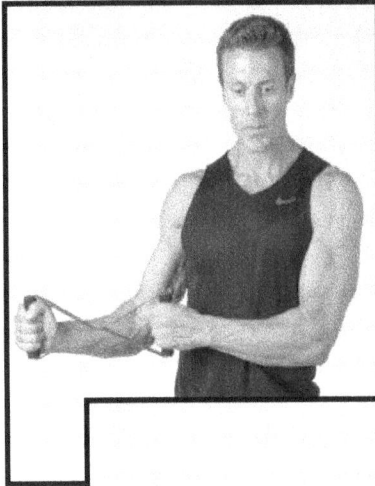
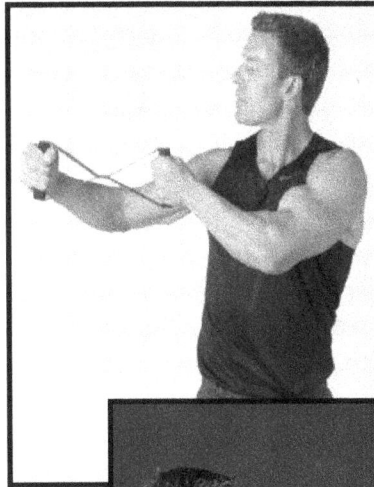
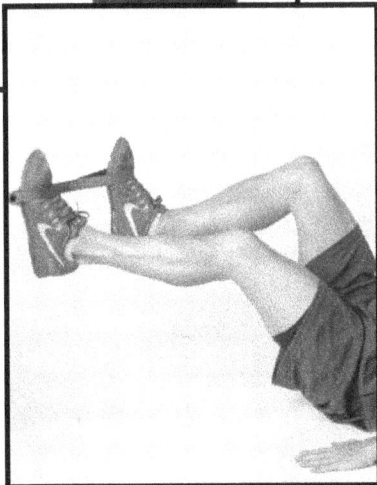
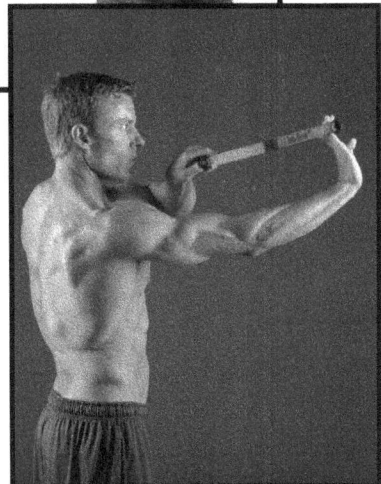

MAX PUMP X1 PROGRAM

13 PHASE ONE

HOW TO PERFORM THIS ROUTINE:
WEEK ONE: 18 Reps per exercise
WEEK TWO: 25 Reps per exercise
WEEK THREE: 5-6 Reps per exercise
**PERFORM A ISOMETRIC CONTRACTION AT THE HALF WAY MARK FOR 5-7 SECONDS
AT THE END OF THE WORK SET. PERFORM 1-2 CIRCUITS**

DAY TWO continued......

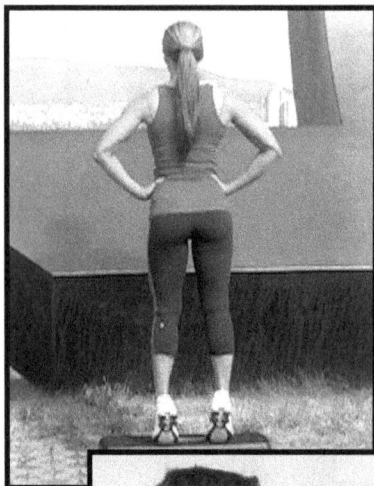

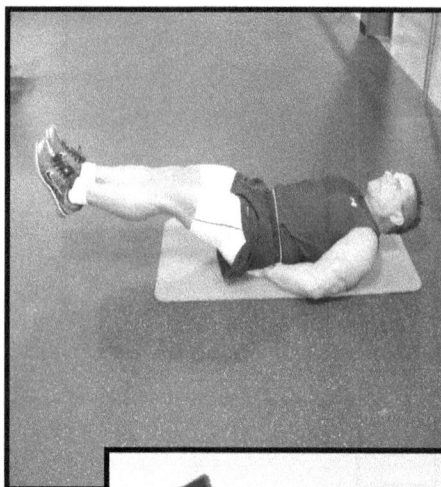

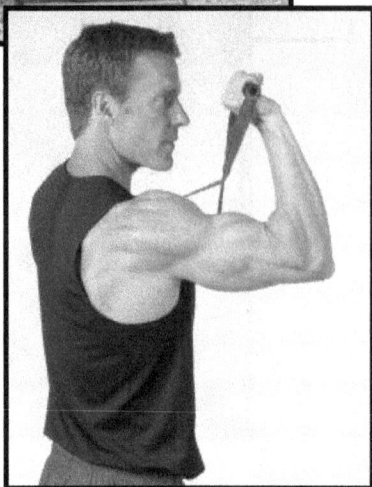

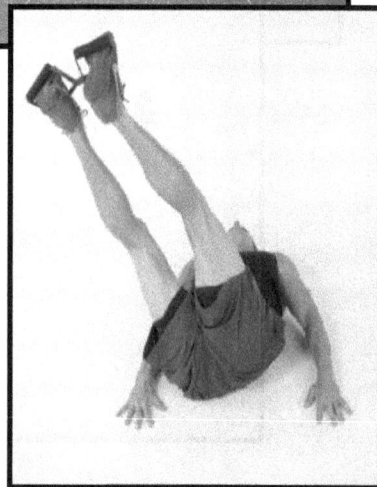

MAX PUMP X1 PROGRAM

13 PHASE ONE

HOW TO PERFORM THIS ROUTINE:
WEEK ONE: 18 Reps per exercise
WEEK TWO: 25 Reps per exercise
WEEK THREE: 5-6 Reps per exercise
**PERFORM A ISOMETRIC CONTRACTION AT THE HALF WAY MARK FOR 5-7 SECONDS
AT THE END OF THE WORK SET. PERFORM 1-2 CIRCUITS**

DAY THREE

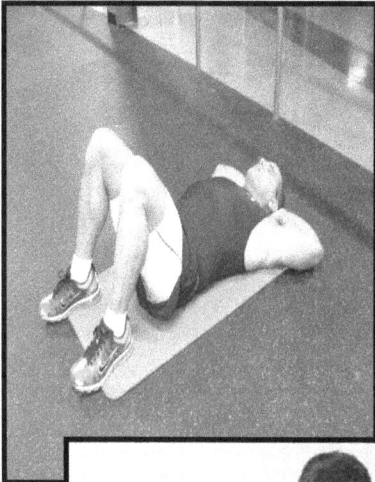
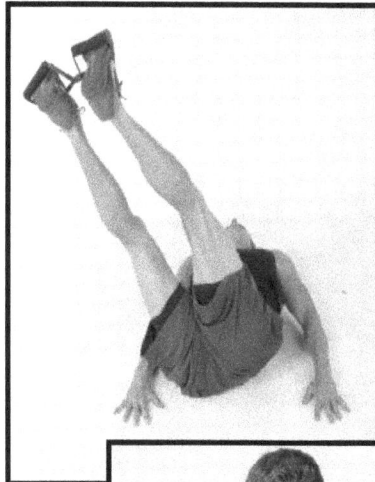
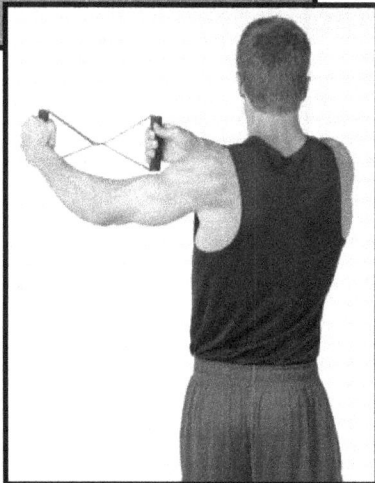
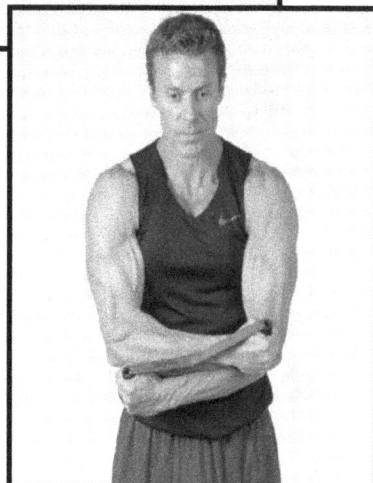

MAX PUMP X1 PROGRAM

13 PHASE ONE

HOW TO PERFORM THIS ROUTINE:
WEEK ONE: 18 Reps per exercise
WEEK TWO: 25 Reps per exercise
WEEK THREE: 5-6 Reps per exercise
**PERFORM A ISOMETRIC CONTRACTION AT THE HALF WAY MARK FOR 5-7 SECONDS
AT THE END OF THE WORK SET. PERFORM 1-2 CIRCUITS**

DAY THREE continued.........

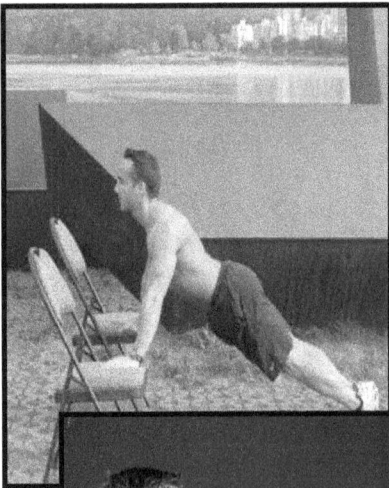

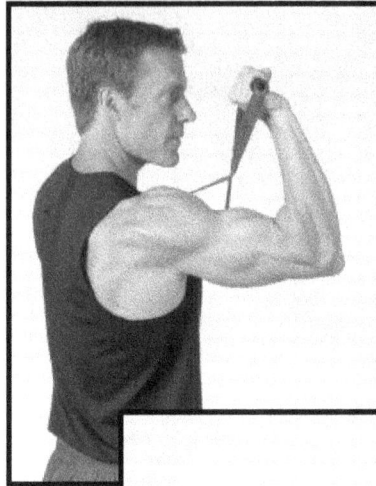

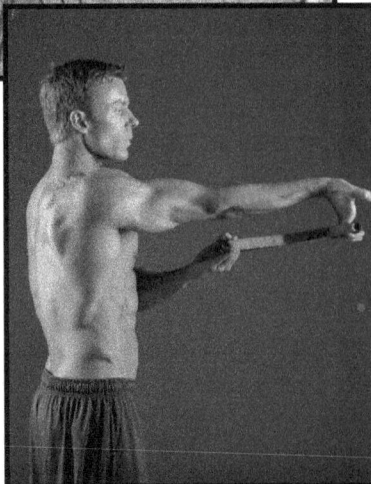

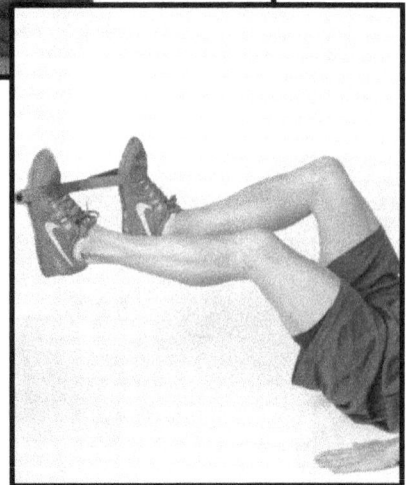

MAX PUMP X1 PROGRAM

13 PHASE ONE

HOW TO PERFORM THIS ROUTINE:

WEEK ONE: 18 Reps per exercise
WEEK TWO: 25 Reps per exercise
WEEK THREE: 5-6 Reps per exercise
PERFORM A ISOMETRIC CONTRACTION AT THE HALF WAY MARK FOR 5-7 SECONDS AT THE END OF THE WORK SET. PERFORM 1-2 CIRCUITS

DAY FOUR

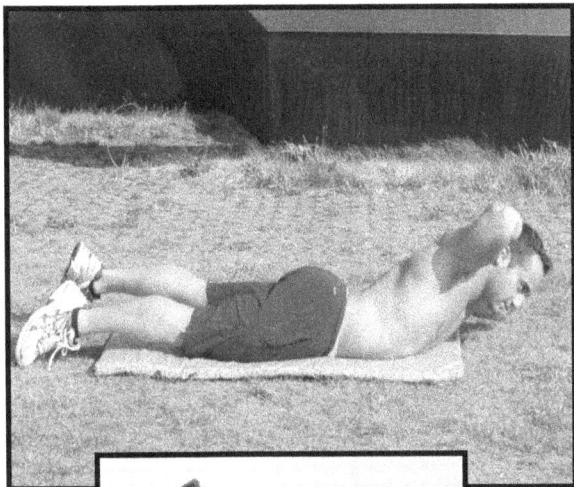
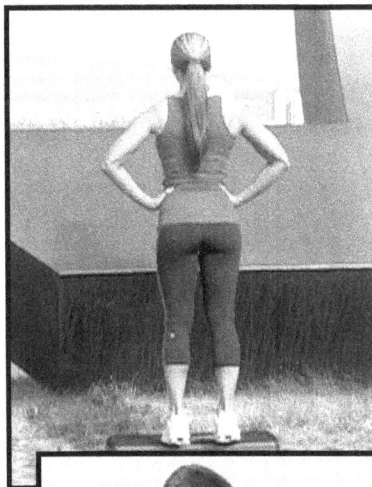
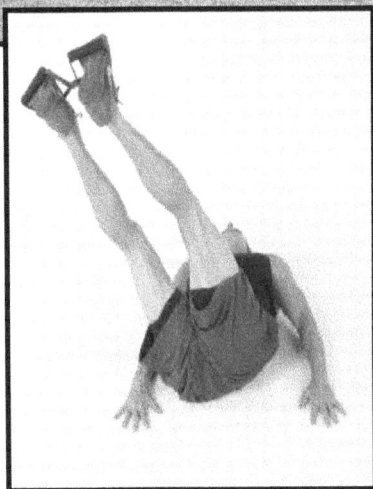
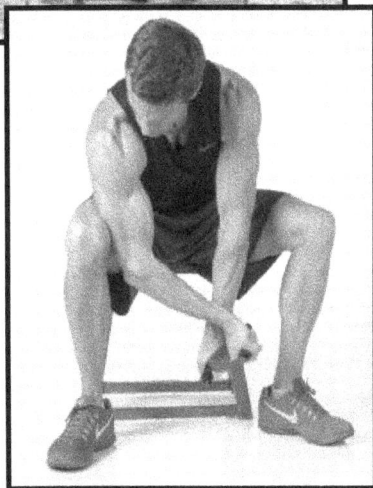

MAX PUMP X1 PROGRAM

13 PHASE ONE

HOW TO PERFORM THIS ROUTINE:
WEEK ONE: 18 Reps per exercise
WEEK TWO: 25 Reps per exercise
WEEK THREE: 5-6 Reps per exercise
PERFORM A ISOMETRIC CONTRACTION AT THE HALF WAY MARK FOR 5-7 SECONDS AT THE END OF THE WORK SET. PERFORM 1-2 CIRCUITS

DAY FIVE

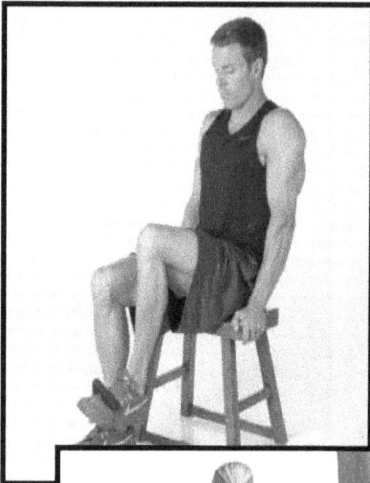

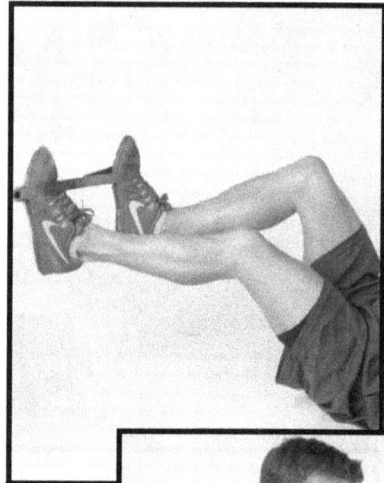

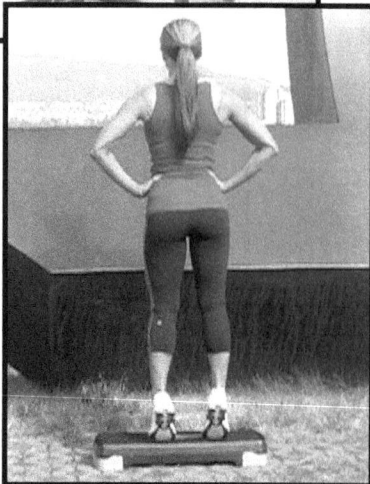

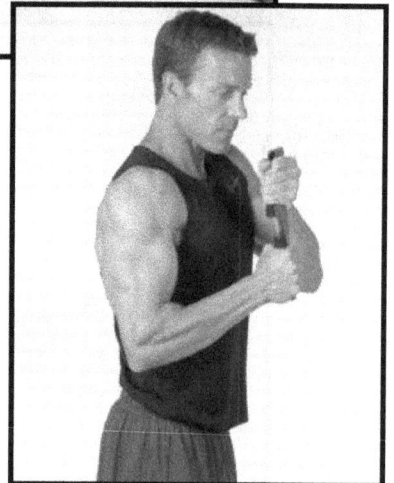

MAX PUMP X1 PROGRAM

13 PHASE ONE

HOW TO PERFORM THIS ROUTINE:
WEEK ONE: 18 Reps per exercise
WEEK TWO: 25 Reps per exercise
WEEK THREE: 5-6 Reps per exercise
PERFORM A ISOMETRIC CONTRACTION AT THE HALF WAY MARK FOR 5-7 SECONDS
AT THE END OF THE WORK SET. PERFORM 1-2 CIRCUITS

DAY FIVE continued............

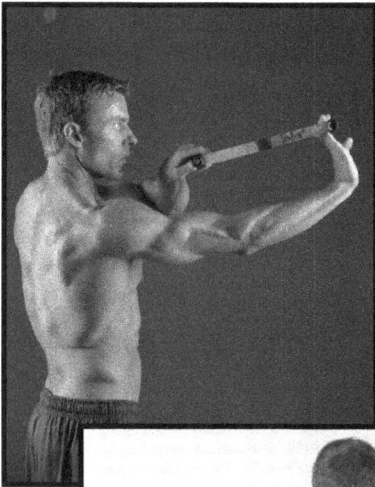

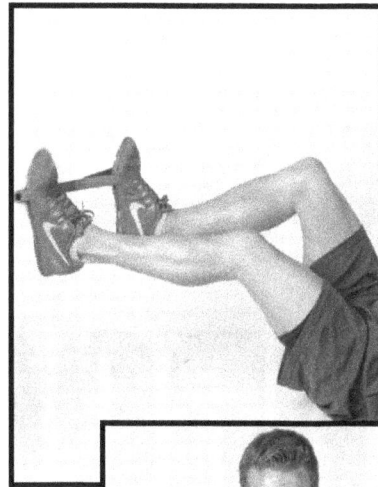

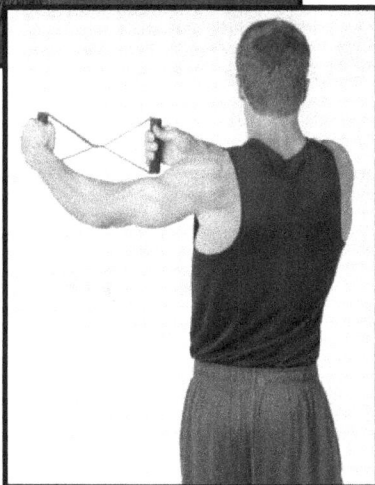

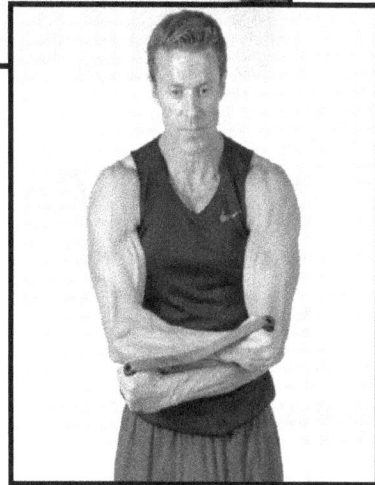

Chapter 13:

THE POWER PUMP MUSCLE-UP PX1 PROGRAM PHASE TWO

REP SPEED 2 SECONDS CONTRACTED, 4 SECONDS RELEASE

THE POWER PUMP MUSCLE-UP PX1 PROGRAM

13 PHASE TWO

HOW TO PERFORM THIS ROUTINE:
PHASE TWO

Perform 7 reps. On the 7th perform an isometric hold for 7 seconds, followed by another 7 reps. Alternate day one and day two for 6 days per week.
PERFORM 1-2 CIRCUITS

DAY ONE

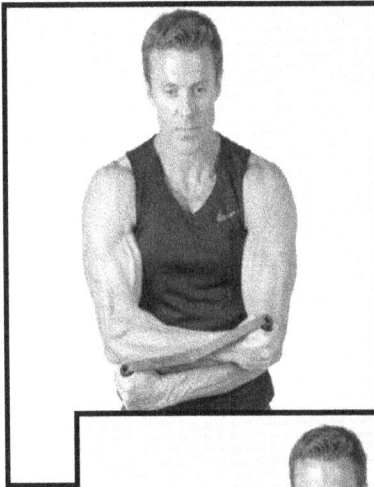
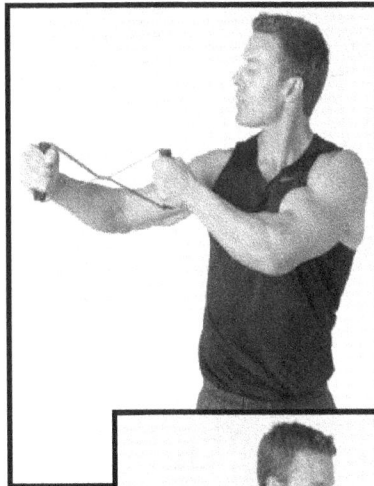
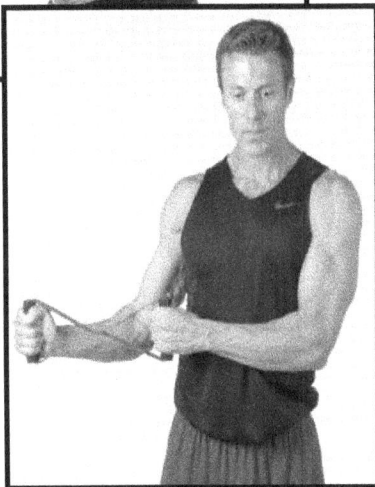
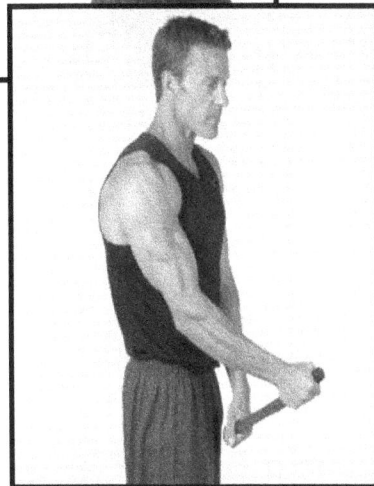

THE POWER PUMP MUSCLE-UP PX1 PROGRAM

13 PHASE TWO

HOW TO PERFORM THIS ROUTINE:
PHASE TWO
Perform 7 reps. On the 7th perform an isometric hold for 7 seconds, followed by another 7 reps. Alternate day one and day two for 6 days per week.
PERFORM 1-2 CIRCUITS

DAY ONE continued..........

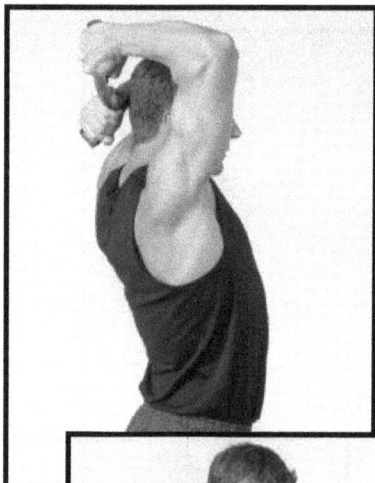

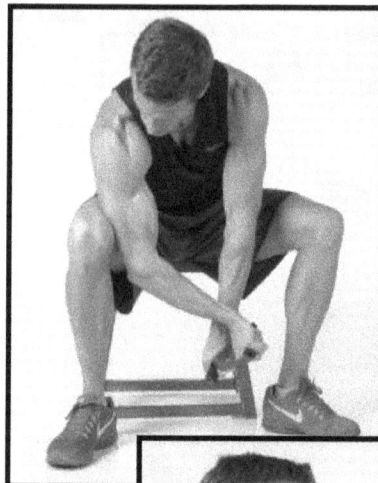

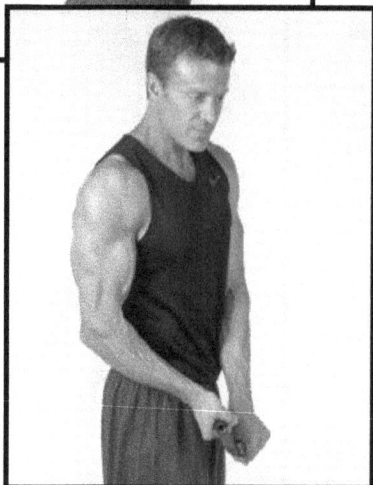

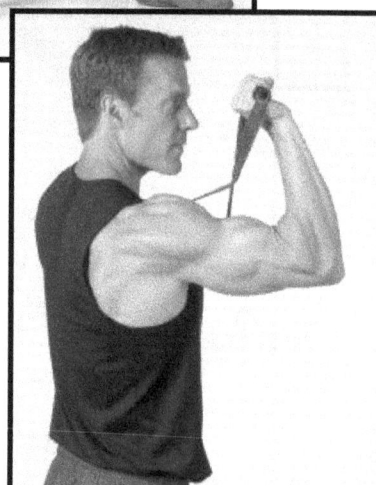

THE POWER PUMP MUSCLE-UP PX1 PROGRAM

13 PHASE TWO

HOW TO PERFORM THIS ROUTINE:
PHASE TWO

Perform 7 reps. On the 7th perform an isometric hold for 7 seconds, followed by another 7 reps. Alternate day one and day two for 6 days per week.
PERFORM 1-2 CIRCUITS

DAY TWO

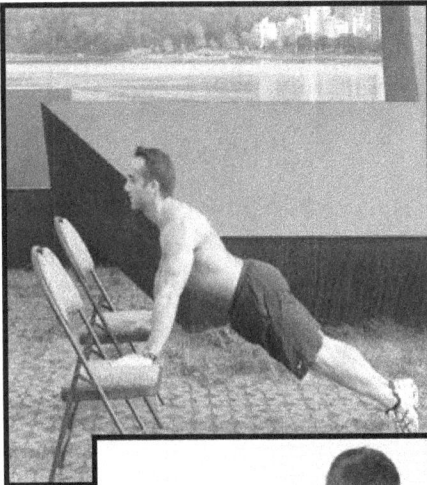
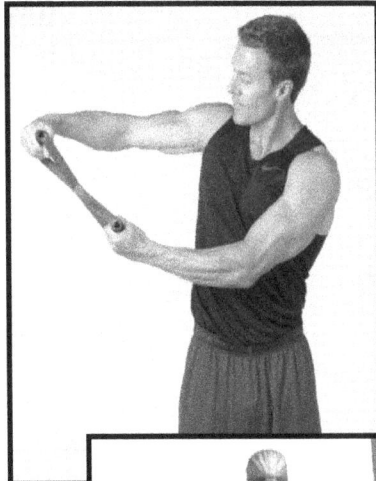
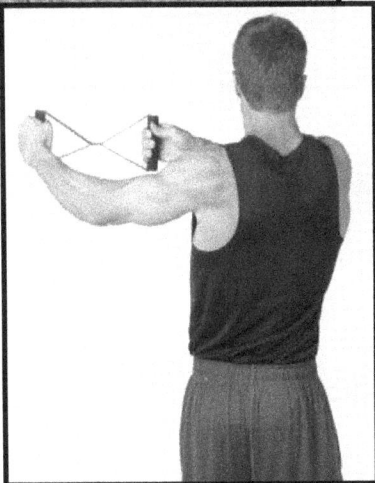
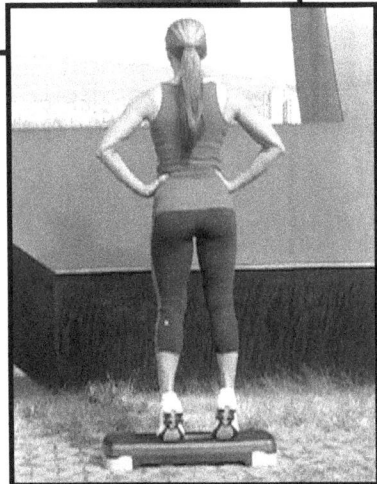

THE POWER PUMP MUSCLE-UP PX1 PROGRAM

13 PHASE TWO

HOW TO PERFORM THIS ROUTINE:
PHASE TWO
Perform 7 reps. On the 7th perform an isometric hold for 7 seconds, followed by another 7 reps. Alternate day one and day two for 6 days per week.
PERFORM 1-2 CIRCUITS

DAY TWO continued........

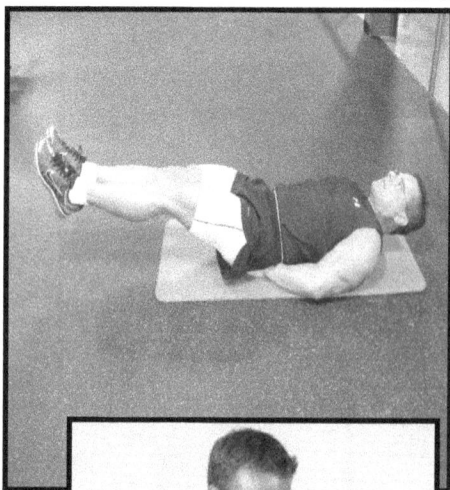
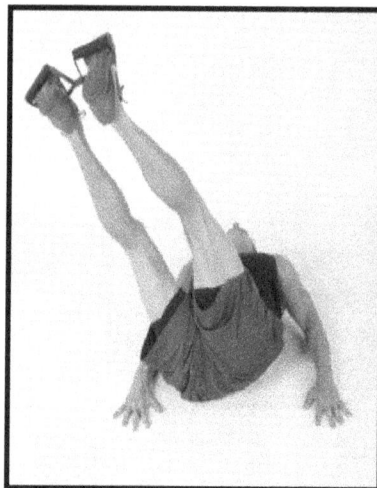
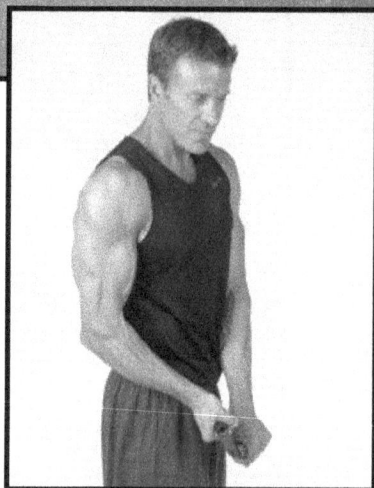
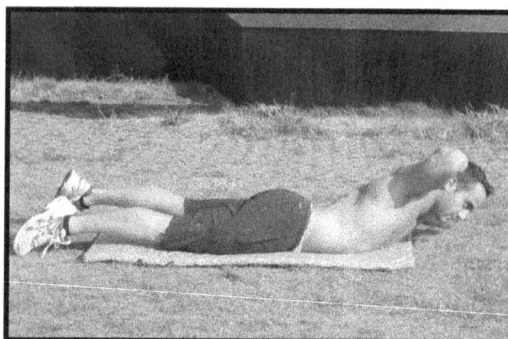

Chapter 13:

THE POWER PUMP MUSCLE-UP PX2 PROGRAM PHASE THREE

REP SPEED 2 SECONDS CONTRACTED, 2 SECONDS RELEASE

THE POWER PUMP MUSCLE-UP PX2 PROGRAM

13 PHASE THREE

HOW TO PERFORM THIS ROUTINE:

Perform 20 reps — On the 20th rep perform a 5 second Isometric hold at the mid-point. Alternate day one and day two for 6 days per week.
PERFORM 1-2 CIRCUITS

DAY ONE

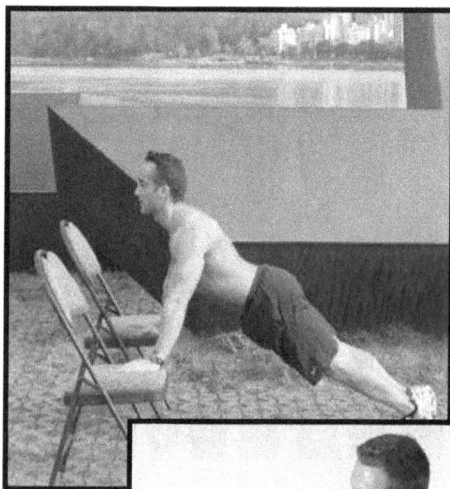
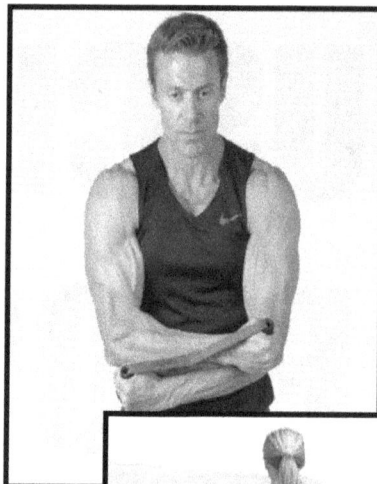
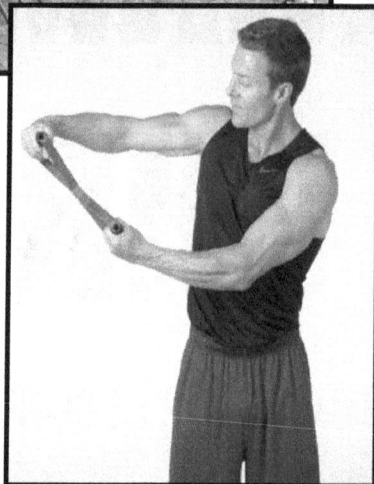
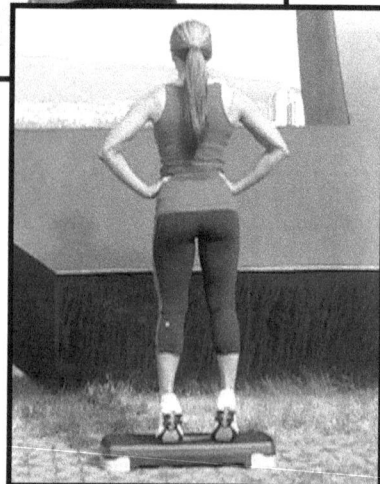

THE POWER PUMP MUSCLE-UP PX2 PROGRAM

13 PHASE THREE

HOW TO PERFORM THIS ROUTINE:

Perform 20 reps — On the 20th rep perform a 5 second Isometric hold at the mid-point. Alternate day one and day two for 6 days per week.
PERFORM 1-2 CIRCUITS

DAY ONE continued...........

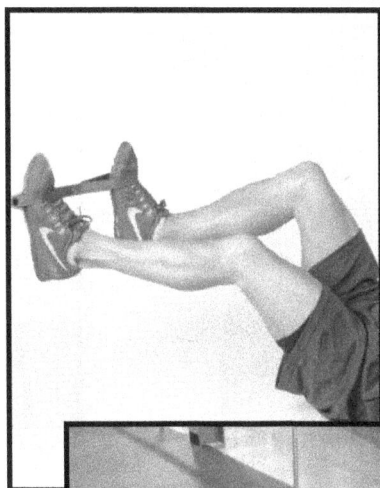

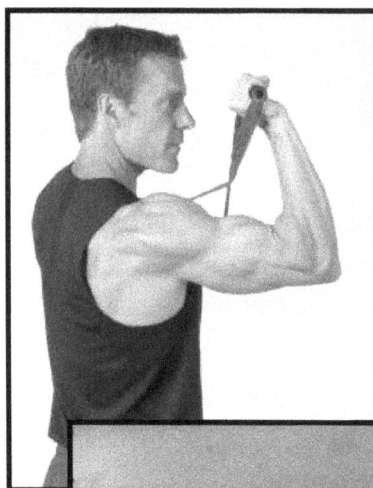

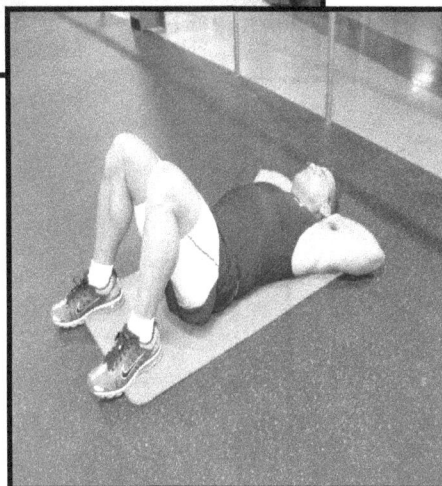

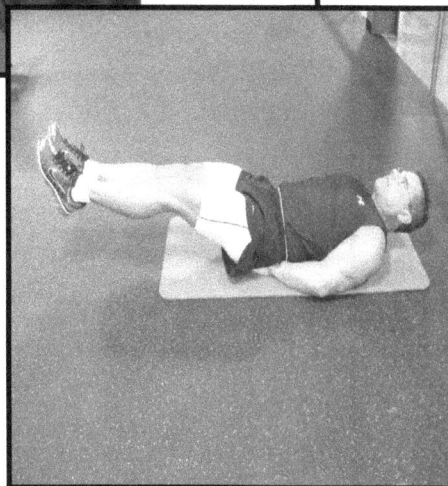

THE POWER PUMP MUSCLE-UP PX2 PROGRAM

13 PHASE THREE

HOW TO PERFORM THIS ROUTINE:

Perform 20 reps — On the 20th rep perform a 5 second Isometric hold at the mid-point. Alternate day one and day two for 6 days per week.
PERFORM 1-2 CIRCUITS

DAY TWO

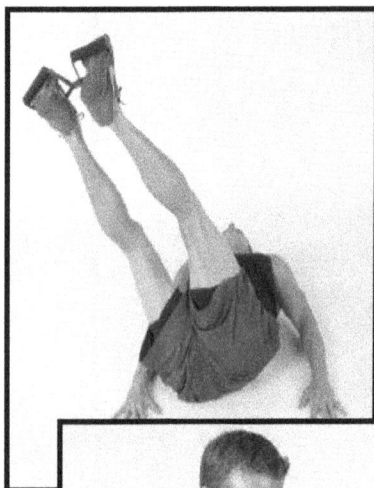
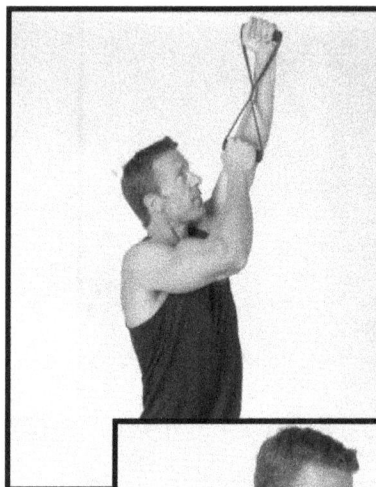
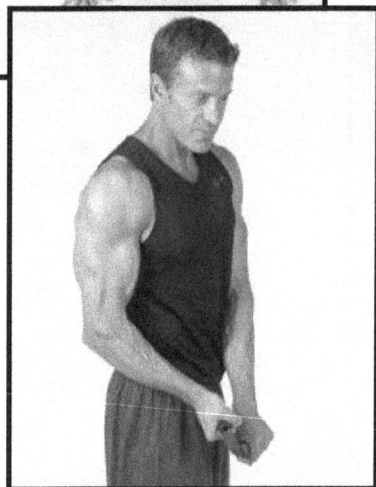
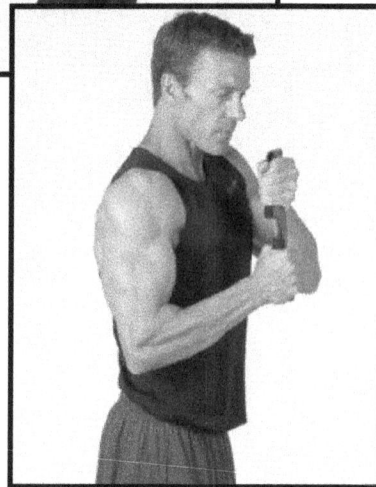

THE POWER PUMP MUSCLE-UP PX2 PROGRAM

13 PHASE THREE

HOW TO PERFORM THIS ROUTINE:
Perform 20 reps — On the 20th rep perform a 5 second Isometric hold at the mid-point. Alternate day one and day two for 6 days per week.
PERFORM 1-2 CIRCUITS

DAY TWO continued..........

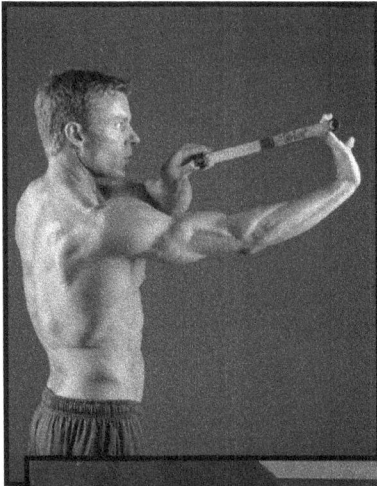

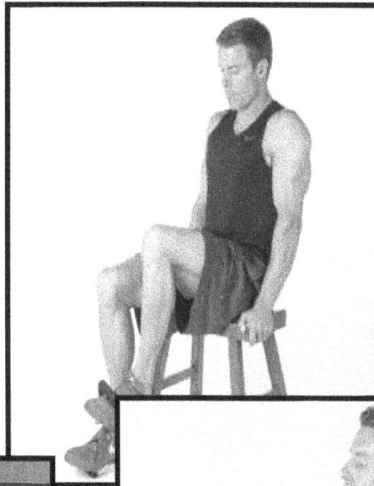

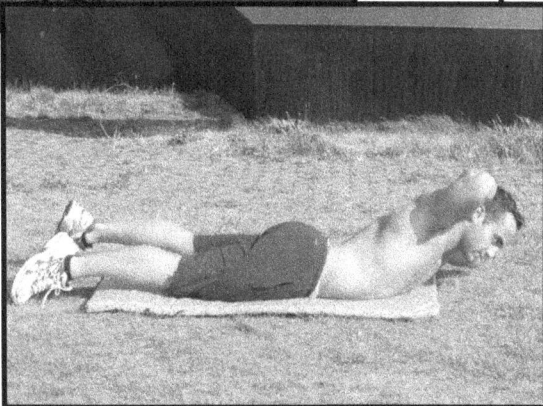

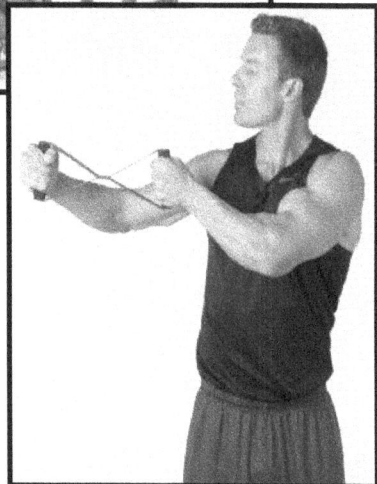

We are looking forward to hearing from you on your progress. Please drop us an email skippymarl@icloud. com

www.ingramcontent.com/pod-product-compliance
Lightning Source LLC
Chambersburg PA
CBHW081159270326
41930CB00014B/3220